A Cree Healer
and His Medicine Bundle

A Cree Healer
and His Medicine Bundle

Revelations of Indigenous Wisdom

HEALING PLANTS, PRACTICES, AND STORIES

David Young, Robert Rogers, and Russell Willier

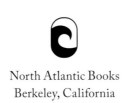

North Atlantic Books
Berkeley, California

Published by   Cover photos by David Young and Robert Rogers
North Atlantic Books   Cover design by Brad Greene
Berkeley, California   Interior design by Jasmine Hromjak

About the cover photos: The pipe, Sweet Grass, and sweat lodge are Lakota, and the shaman's drum is Dogrib Dene from the Northwest Territories. Depicted at the bottom, from top left are Prairie Sage, Labrador Tea, and Sweet Grass; at the very bottom are White Sage (*Artemisia ludoviciana*), Reindeer Moss, and Yarrow.

Maps used by permission of Backroad Mapbooks
Printed in the United States of America

Disclaimer: This book is not in any way intended to replace the services of a licensed health-care provider in the diagnosis or treatment of illness or disease. Any application of the material in the following pages is at the reader's discretion.

A Cree Healer and His Medicine Bundle: Revelations of Indigenous Wisdom—Healing Plants, Practices, and Stories is sponsored and published by the Society for the Study of Native Arts and Sciences (dba North Atlantic Books), an educational nonprofit based in Berkeley, California, that collaborates with partners to develop cross-cultural perspectives, nurture holistic views of art, science, the humanities, and healing, and seed personal and global transformation by publishing work on the relationship of body, spirit, and nature.

North Atlantic Books' publications are available through most bookstores. For further information, visit our website at www.northatlanticbooks.com or call 800-733-3000.

Library of Congress Cataloging-in-Publication Data

Young, David E. (David Earl)
  A Cree healer and his medicine bundle : revelations of indigenous wisdom / David Young, Robert Rogers, Russell Willier.
    pages   cm
  ISBN 978-1-58394-903-0 (paperback) — ISBN 978-1-58394-904-7 (ebook)
  1. Willier, Russell. 2. Willier, Russell—Philosophy. 3. Cree Indians—Biography. 4. Shamans—Alberta—Biography. 5. Medicinal plants—Alberta. 6. Cree Indians—Medicine. 7. Traditional medicine—Alberta. I. Rogers, Robert Dale, 1950– II. Willier, Russell. III. Title.
  E99.C88Y68 2015
  971.2004'97323092—dc23
  [B]

                                  2014024236

            3 4 5 6 7 8 9 VERSA 21 20 19 18 17

This book is dedicated to the numerous Native healers who have suffered so much discrimination in the past and who continue to dedicate their lives to helping aboriginal peoples and to preserving traditional medicinal knowledge.

Acknowledgments

We would like to thank the Canadian Circumpolar Institute and the Centre for the Cross-Cultural Study of Health and Healing (now the Centre for Health and Culture) at the University of Alberta for funding the fieldwork upon which this book is founded. We would also like to thank Clifford Cardinal for providing the correct orthography for the Cree terms Russell Willier uses for his medicinal plants, as well as Mussio Ventures Ltd. for allowing us to use maps from their *Backroad Mapbook* of northern Alberta. We are grateful to Nancy Turner for providing corrections.

Contents

Preface

David Young

I first encountered aboriginal religion and medicine in 1984 when I participated in a multidisciplinary project to document the traditional skin-tanning methods of Russell and Yvonne Willier on the Sucker Creek Reserve in northern Alberta. In the course of getting to know the Williers, I was surprised to learn that Russell Willier is a Cree healer. As a result of our growing friendship, Russell developed a degree of trust that allowed him to talk about his beliefs and practices in a way that he was not accustomed to doing with outsiders. This trust was further enhanced when I described my own background in Zen Buddhism, which seemed to Russell to be quite compatible with many of his own beliefs and practices.

At the conclusion of the skin-tanning project, a new project (Project for the Study of Traditional Healing Practices) was set up as a multidisciplinary effort involving anthropologists at the University of Alberta, graduate students in the Department of Anthropology at the University of Alberta, Dr. Janice Morse from the Faculty of Nursing at the University of Alberta, individuals from the Provincial Museum of Alberta (now the Royal Alberta Museum), the Boyle McCauley Clinic in Edmonton, and Dr. Steven Aung. The project was made possible by a research grant from the University of Alberta. Research associated with the Project for the Study of Traditional Healing Practices, which spanned a five-year period, consisted of conducting fieldwork on the Sucker Creek Reserve in northern Alberta, helping Russell Willier collect wild plants for his medicines, participating in ceremonies, and documenting the progress of several non-Native patients who were treated by Russell for psoriasis. The results of this research are summarized in a book, *Cry of the Eagle: Encounters with a Cree Healer* (1989), and in a variety of journal articles.

In 1985, our interdisciplinary team documented Russell Willier treating ten non-Native patients with psoriasis, recruited through advertisements in a local paper. Psoriasis is an itchy, scaly skin disease that affects 2 to 6 percent of the world's population. Although Russell Willier treats a variety of diseases, we selected psoriasis for treatment because it is highly visible and the effects of treatment can easily be monitored. The experiment consisted of two stages. In the first stage, patients were treated in the Boyle McCauley Clinic, a downtown Edmonton facility where doctors and nurses could observe the process. In the second stage, patients participated in sweat lodge ceremonies on an acreage near Edmonton. The healer came to Edmonton periodically over a period of several months. Treatment at the clinic consisted of purifying the room and other religious ceremonies, followed by having patients drink an herbal tea, after which a solution containing a number of ingredients was applied to the skin of the patients. Documentation included video footage, still photographs, and tracing the outline of major lesions on transparent material to provide a record of change in size of the lesions over time. Sweat lodge ceremonies involved constructing a sweat lodge on the first day of the ceremony. Patients arrived around three in the afternoon. Dressed in swimsuits or loose-fitting gowns, patients sat in a circle inside the sweat lodge, around a pit filled with red-hot rocks. After the entrance was closed, the healer prayed, chanted, and talked while sprinkling herbal water on the rocks to create a hot steam. The "sweat" consisted of four rounds, with each round lasting about half an hour. This part of the experiment consisted of three sweat lodge ceremonies for patients, followed by a fourth ceremony for spouses and children. Following the final sweat, a thanking ceremony was held to thank the spirits for assisting.

Patients had a variety of experiences during the ceremonies, such as hearing the cry of an eagle and seeing moving lights. In many cases, psoriasis lesions peeled off as a result of the heat and moisture. A month later, patients met for the last time at the clinic so a physician could evaluate their progress. Six patients were considered significantly improved. One of these made a full recovery from psoriasis on his hands. The other four, despite earlier improvement, had reverted to their original conditions. Though the research team considered the results significant, Willier was disappointed and said that if he were to treat any further patients, it would have to be at his reserve, where the process would be conducted in a more traditional manner. The results of treating two teenagers at the reserve are described in Part III, "The Efficacy of Native Medicine."

While working with Russell Willier, there were two occasions on which our research team was invited to accompany Willier on expeditions to collect herbs. The first trip was conducted from June 15 to 18, 1985, in the Grouard, Alberta, area. A supplemental field trip was taken from August 31 to September 2, 1985, during which additional medicinal plants were collected and identified. Original identification of most of the plants in Russell Willier's herbal repertoire was done by Judith Golub, who also collected plant specimens for the museum. Most of the photos on the original field trip were taken by Ruth McConnell. There were several plants collected whose identification was unclear. Robert Rogers, assistant clinical professor in the Department of Family Medicine at the University of Alberta and a well-known herbalist who has authored several books on medicinal plants, has identified these plants for the present book. He also identified several new plants that Russell has added to his repertoire since the 1985 fieldwork.

After retiring and moving to Japan, I lost touch with Russell Willier until 2010, when the Centre for the Cross-Cultural Study of Health and Healing at the University of Alberta convened a conference of Native healers to address the issue of how to preserve traditional medicinal knowledge when so many elders are dying without passing on their knowledge. Although I was unable to attend the conference, I requested that Russell Willier be invited to the conference. While in attendance at the conference, Russell met two delegates from the Vancouver area, one of whom, Don Gatley, subsequently invited Russell Willier to visit the island of Gabriola. This gave Russell and me the opportunity to resume working together, one result of which is the publication of this book featuring Russell's medicine bundle. The original manuscript for the book *Cry of the Eagle: Encounters with a Cree Healer* contained a chapter on Russell's herbal repertoire, but we decided to remove it prior to publication due to substantial opposition from members of the Native community as well as members of the Western medical community. At that time, the Native community was opposed to sharing information with outsiders, because Europeans had stolen so much from them and they were determined not to have their religion and medicine stolen as well. The Western medical community was also suspicious of Native medicine, believing it to be unscientific and based upon superstition. At one point in our research, the Dean of the Faculty of Medicine at the University of Alberta summoned me to his office to show me a letter he had received from a prominent physician in Edmonton who was demanding to know why the university was funding research on witch doctors.

Russell's hope of building a traditional healing center on his reserve had never materialized. Although government money was made available to the band council, it was used to construct a nursing station that was later turned into a day care establishment. After that, Russell gave up on the center, until recently when his hopes were rekindled by his contact with Don Gatley, mentioned above. Don and a group of his associates are considering the possibility of building a healing center on land owned by Don and his wife, Glenna Borsuk, on Gabriola Island, off the coast of British Columbia. Situated on this land are ancient burial caves and petroglyphs, including a rock carving of the Mouse Woman, a Grandmother (Spirit Helper) responsible for helping young people to whom an injustice has been done. She also is a healer. Russell has brought several people to the sacred site, where they have been healed from a variety of ailments. I have documented this process in a monograph: *The Mouse Woman of Gabriola: Brain, Mind, and Icon Interactions in Spontaneous Healing* (Young 2013).

There have also been major changes in the relations between Native and Western medicine. Over the years, as Native healers, both men and women, continued to die without passing on their knowledge of traditional medicine, it became apparent that Native medicine could die out and that it needed the help of researchers if it were to survive. In 2009, a Native healer, Clifford Cardinal, was given an academic appointment in the Department of Family Medicine at the University of Alberta, with a joint appointment in the Centre for the Cross-Cultural Study of Health and Healing. He spends part of his time lecturing to medical students on Native medicine; Clifford is also enrolled in a PhD program in Mind Body Medicine with HMS University. It was Clifford Cardinal and Earle

Waugh, director of the Centre for Health and Culture at the University of Alberta (formerly the Centre for the Cross-Cultural Study of Health and Healing), who organized the gathering of healers at the university in 2010 to consider ways to preserve Native medicine for future generations. There was general agreement at this gathering that traditional medicinal knowledge should be written down and documented in such a fashion that it would not be lost in the future.

A major problem remains: how to document traditional medicine without giving the knowledge to pharmaceutical companies who would employ this knowledge for profit by creating drugs that would be used in a non-ritual context. The result is the present book, in which we document individual plants and how they are used, without publishing the complex combinations that are used for healing difficult cases. The book will aid, however, in passing on these combinations, as a healer will be able to instruct apprentices by saying, for example, that for heart problems, combine the plants on pages 55, 58, 62, 64, and 71 (note: not an actual formula). This formula would be accompanied by information concerning when to collect the herbs, how to combine them, and how to preserve them. The intent of the book is to provide photographs that are sufficiently clear to allow the plants to be identified and collected in their natural habitats as a way to help preserve Native medicine for the future. In addition to making a contribution to the preservation of indigenous medical knowledge, the book should be of interest to indigenous people in general, those interested in natural healing, herbalists, ethnobotanists, and medicine hunters in general, as well as those interested in boreal forest plants. It may also appeal to naturopaths, and complementary and alternative health practitioners, including medical doctors, chiropractors, and other healing professionals. Finally, the book should be useful to ethnologists, anthropologists, and those teaching in medical schools, social science departments, and Native Studies departments in colleges and universities.

I have edited the material provided by Russell Willier in the first four chapters, and have written the material on Russell Willier in Chapter Five, Part III on the efficacy of Native medicine, and the Conclusion. Robert Rogers has supplied the additional material for Chapter Five.

Part I

Russell Willier, Cree Healer

In the Preface, David Young briefly described the events leading up to the publication of this book. In Part I, Russell Willier speaks for himself, discussing how he became a healer, his life as a healer, his beliefs about the universe, and the ecological issues of importance to his role as a medicine person. He also relates several of his favorite "healing stories." Some of this material takes the form of interviews that have been only slightly edited. The goal is to let Russell Willier's personality shine through, something that tends to be lost in academic writing. Part II will present Russell Willier's medicine bundle—his repertoire of plants used in his healing practice.

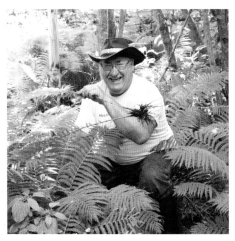

Russell Willier picking *Dryopteris carthusiana*
(Photo by David Young)

Chapter One

Willier's Life as a Healer

Becoming a Medicine Man

I had to learn from the older people, plus when I was a little boy, I was the one to dig different herbs for the old ladies. They would show me which herbs they wanted. They would offer some tobacco, watch, and pray, while I collected the herbs. I would bring all the herbs to the old ladies who were sitting there cleaning them. They didn't go from one herb to the next, kneeling down; they were just sitting there. It was the same with my mom, my aunties, and some other old ladies who were the medicine men's wives. After a few years, I started to understand which herbs they wanted without them telling me, and which areas the herbs were in. That's one of the reasons I want to have photographs of the areas where herbs are found in this book, because you can just about rake the whole of Alberta before you find the herb you are looking for unless you know the kind of area it is in. People figure it's just in the bush. It's not just in the bush. On the trip we just finished, we had to go 1,000 kilometers to see the majority of the plants that I use. Even so, we had to know exactly where to look. All the books that I've seen have the same problem: they have a beautiful picture of the plant and they write down where you find it. But once you're out in the bush, it doesn't look the same as what you've been reading.

My medicine bundle came from my great-grandfather, Moostoos, a famous medicine man who signed Treaty 8 for our area. The bundle was given to my father and passed on to me when I was about nineteen or twenty years old. At first I didn't want to use it, as I didn't want to be a medicine man. As the years went by, when I was around thirty, different medicine men knew they were going to die. Also some of the old ladies I had helped said they might not make it through this winter.

So they started looking around; they couldn't pass their knowledge on to their grandchildren or their children because they were on drugs or drunk. They couldn't give it to them even if they wanted to. So they decided they had better give it to me. When one person would tell me how to use a certain herb or combination, I then had to ask, "How do I know if it's any good? I don't want to doctor somebody and use this combination and find out it doesn't do any good." So what the medicine people told me was: "Come and watch us doctoring and then if you want to use the combination, go check on the individual six weeks to three months later. They will tell you how they're doing." When I did that, one of the patients I visited might say, "Oh, I ended up with a doctor." Right away I would cross that combination off, since it didn't help that individual. You wouldn't believe how many combinations there are across Canada. You have to select the best ones, the ones that will work right away. I went and watched people get doctored; then six weeks later I was at their door. I told them I was checking up on them because the old man, my teacher, couldn't come. If they said, "I got all better. My legs don't hurt anymore and my back is good," I knew I could use that combination on someone with a similar problem. Then you get into the spiritual world. A lot of times the spirits tell you to use a particular combination. You don't select it; you are told what to use. You don't question it. But if the combination is passed on from a human, you really have to check. Don't trust any individual. Check it out for yourself.

When I first opened the medicine bundle, I didn't know what the herbs tied together in little bundles were used for, so I had to go to different medicine people to see if they knew how to use the combinations in the medicine bundle. Some combinations were wrapped in individual pieces of rawhide. The original medicine bundle was moose skin. I don't have it anymore. My house burned down, so I lost everything, but I already knew the combinations by then. What we're trying to do here with this book is to pass the same combinations on with pictures. They didn't have that.

I doctored lots in the 1980s and '90s. If you're a medicine person, you can't keep a regular nine to five job. If you want to be a medicine person, you have to take small contracts from three days to a week and not much more—working on a fence or trap line. You get a few dollars. You need this money because when you doctor, you can't ask for money. It's up to the individual. I went quite a few times to Valleyview or Edmonton. I do get the tobacco, but beyond that I often don't get enough to buy gas there and back. A lot of people don't have any consideration. People should go out and do the 1,000 kilometers picking herbs. It would teach them to respect how much work it is to collect the plants you need.

Approaching a Healer

The proper way to approach me and other Cree healers is to present me with a square meter of cotton cloth: white, yellow, red, blue, or green (see the Medicine Wheel diagram on the following page), a pouch of unflavored pipe tobacco, and a gift. The individual making the request decides which color of cloth to present. I then compare the color of the cloth presented with the color of the individual's aura, as different colors are associated with different diseases and illnesses. After receiving a request for help, I have four choices: if I have treated this particular problem successfully before, I may give a positive response without delay; if I have never treated the problem, I may tell the individual that I will need several days to meditate and pray—asking the spirits whether I should take on this case; I may refer the patient to another healer known for treating this particular problem; or I may tell the person to see a medical doctor without delay, as in the case of a severe infection. If I choose to meditate and pray, I do so in the bush; if I am instructed by the spirits to treat the patient, I seek a vision in which one of the Grandfather spirits appears to me to provide me with instructions concerning which plants (and possibly animal parts or minerals) to use, where to find them if I do not already know, and how to combine the ingredients.

The cloth and tobacco presented to me are used when treating patients individually or in ceremonies such as the sweat lodge or sun dance ceremony. Tobacco is offered when the first plant of a specific species is collected for medicine, when the first rock is taken for the sweat lodge ceremony, or when willow boughs are cut for constructing a sweat lodge. Tobacco is also sprinkled around a sweat lodge to provide protection from evil spirits. Tobacco is used in numerous other ways.

My Cosmology

My beliefs about the world are shown in the following Medicine Wheel diagram, in which a number of different variables are systematically related. For example, the direction East is associated with the Sun, the Eagle spirit, Autumn, and the color yellow. The circumference of the circle represents the Sweetgrass Trail, around which the individual travels as he seeks to pass through life successfully and eventually return to the Great Spirit, the source of all life. This diagram does not attempt to be all-inclusive, rather, it provides examples of the kinds of factors and forces that play a role in how the world is ordered. The complex nature of their relationships must be understood by anyone, such as a healer, who seeks to tap in to the wisdom and power of the Cosmos.

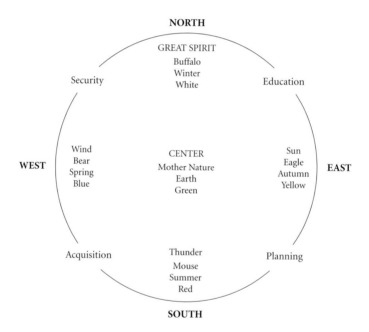

The hierarchical nature of the Cosmos, especially as it pertains to healing, is shown in the following diagram.

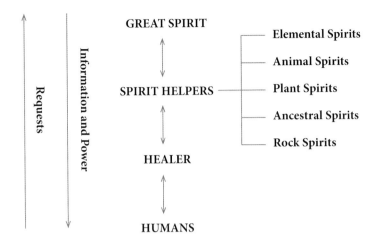

The primary role of a healer is to help people who approach him in the correct way, asking for healing and guidance from the Great Spirit. Since the Great Spirit is too holy to be approached directly, the healer must work with Spirit Helpers, the Grandfathers. The Grandfathers carry requests from the healer to the Great Spirit and return to the healer with information and spiritual power. The healer then channels this assistance to those who have requested it. In other words, the healer is an intermediary between ordinary humans and Spirit Helpers, who, in turn, are intermediaries between the healer and the Great Spirit.

There are various kinds of Spirit Helpers: elemental spirits representing the primordial forces of Nature such as the Sun, Wind, and Thunder; animal spirits such as Eagle, Bear, and Mouse; and plant spirits such as "Bear Root" (*Aralia nudicaulis,* Wild Sarsaparilla) and "Frog Pants" (*Sarracenia purpurea,* Pitcher Plant). Even objects such as rocks, which most non-Native people consider "inanimate," can be Spirit Helpers. In fact, rocks are some of the most important Grandfather spirits, as they have been here from the beginning of the world and will be here long after people, trees, and plants are gone. The Grandfathers also include the spirits of those individuals who have gone before. Each species of animal, plant, fish, and insect has its own Grandfather spirit, of which all members of that species are living expressions.

The situation is further complicated by the fact that everything that works for the good in the world is duplicated by an equivalent set of spirits that work for the bad. Thus, for example, the good North Wind (a subcategory of Wind, shown in the above cosmology diagram) is countered by a bad North Wind. The only exception to this dualistic worldview is the Great Spirit, which does not have an evil counterpart such as the Devil. In the long run, the Great Spirit will ensure that good wins out over evil; this prevents my belief system from being truly dualistic. In the meantime, however, the battle between good and evil is a real one that impinges in many important ways upon the health of individuals and upon the role of healers. It influences health in that sometimes the physical, spiritual, or emotional problems experienced by individuals are due to curses sent their way by evil healers who are working for the "bad side." Bad healers often respond to requests by individuals who have a grudge against others, in return for substantial sums of money. An important task of a good healer is to diagnose which problems are caused by curses as opposed to problems due to natural causes. When a curse is diagnosed as being the source of the problem, the healer can take ceremonial steps to stop or deflect the curse, sometimes sending it back from where it came. Engaging in this kind of spiritual warfare involves considerable risk for a healer, who may himself become the object of a curse.

Native Medicine

There are many things that I would like to talk to you about to give you a general insight into traditional Native medicine. First, there are a few misunderstandings I would like to clarify. There is really only one God though he has different names such as the Great Spirit, Allah, Buddha, and the Creator. The Creator has many kinds of helpers, such as natural elements (fire, water, thunder, wind), animals, fish, plants, birds, and our loved ones who have passed on before us. We call these helpers Grandmothers and Grandfathers. We believe that God sent these grandparents to help us. We ask them to talk to God for us, because nobody can talk directly to God. We are worth no more than a blade of grass; we are no higher than anything that God has made. Therefore, we humans need someone to take our messages to God for us.

Native people use smudging as a way to purify ourselves in mind, body, and spirit. Materials used for smudging include Sweet Grass, Sage, Cedar, and the Diamond Willow Fungus. When we burn these, the smoke carries our prayers up to the Creator. God gave us plants to use. We use plant combinations that have been around for centuries. In the last century, we have been using Western medicine because the government banned Native medicine. There were times when medicine people had to go underground and hide while they helped people. Many traditional medicines got lost when our children were sent to the residential schools. Other things were lost as well, such as language and family relationships.

Traditionally, Native people were taught that God was a loving and caring entity while the church told them that God was someone to be feared. There was no hell in Native culture, but there was in Western culture. We were told that God could read our thoughts and that Native religion was evil. We were told that we must not ask the spirits for help. Native culture is passed down orally. With the breakdown of family relationships and having to hide our spirituality, many traditions were lost. Medicine people were no longer held in such high regard; they were made out to be the black sheep of society. They could no longer pass their beliefs down to their children and grandchildren. Today, very few people still believe in Native spirituality.

Now you are probably thinking, OK, but that's the past; how does this relate to today's issues? Unfortunately, a lot of the problems from the past are still plaguing people today. Native people need to have their basic needs met: adequate housing, nutritional food, health care, and clean drinking water. Our elders are being ignored. There are still many of them who do not speak English and need interpreters. Elders are this generation's key to our own traditions, but they cannot be heard. There are so many illnesses that are affecting Native people, diabetes and cancer being the major ones. Preventive measures for diabetes need to be taught and enforced in Native communities. Western medicine has become a necessity for surviving. We must find ways to work together to make Canada a healthier place. Things have improved in the last decade or so.

But keep in mind that most of the elders are dead. They went through hell with Western culture and medicine. The new generations

don't speak their language or practice their culture. The younger people have to be treated with Western medicine. There are still a few families who doctor others and practice their spirituality, but people who practice traditional culture are considered the black sheep of the community and are picked on by different religions, especially born-again Christians. The culture itself will eventually die off if things don't turn around soon for Native people.

The Grandfathers and Grandmothers are always there. It doesn't matter what nationality, when you're going to die, your parents are going to be over there whether you believe it or not. Even if you are a nonbeliever, whoever loved you will be there to guide you to the next world. You're not going alone. If that were planted in everybody's head it might help a lot, because those are the same ones we pray to for help. The grandparents are kindhearted. They try to do their best. Recently the elders came to my place and said, "We should have a special ceremony to offer food to those who have died." "Yeah, we will," I said. "No problem." They said that they would get some heart, moose nose, and tongue. I asked, "What do the young people, age thirty and under, like?" They thought about it and said, "Pizza, I guess." I said, "That's what we will put on the fire. We have to go with the world. We shouldn't be stuck in time. If it's a young person who loved pizza, then we feed him pizza."

Collecting Plants

I collect most of my plants in the fall. In late July you can still get some flowering plants, though some of them have already seeded. We take the late-flowering plants because if we collect them in May and June, they don't have a chance to seed and they will get wiped out [when the plants have flowers it makes them easier to identify, even if one is mainly after the roots]. If we're after the roots, we take them in the fall. Including young trees, bark, etc., I mainly use about twenty-eight plants. Some of the plants are hard to get. Plus I use another thirty-three plants on a more occasional basis. Sometimes I have to go a long ways to find my plants. Sometimes they will put a pipeline right through the herbs that you use. They figure the same plants are everywhere. They don't care. Recently I was given permission to pick herbs in the Alberta provincial parks. We had a big meeting. The parks department wanted bigger parks in Alberta. I said we have no problem with that, but we can't pick herbs in the parks. We can get charged if we pick in the parks. We should be allowed to take herbs there. So they agreed that we could take the herbs in any park in Alberta. They said if you go to a park, tell the ranger that you will be taking herbs. They can't stop you. Tell them what plants you will be taking. See, there's a lot of Rat Root and Bear Root in Alert Bay.

It is important to know how plants look in the summer and in the fall when the part above ground is dead. The roots though are still alive, so I usually just take the roots in the fall. But you don't want to take too many. If you see the Morning Flower or Gum Flower here and there, keep driving and look for where they are really thick; then you can take the flowers but leave the roots. I hope everybody does the same. There's not too many flowers that we use, but those are two of them. If I pick plants in the summer, I wait for them to deflower so the seeds get spread, unless I need the flower itself.

When we photographed the plants, I gave you an English name such as Big Arrow. In most books you won't find the name Big Arrow. That is a translation of the Cree word. You have to do this since the Cree language is being lost and the young people won't be able to understand Cree. They will need an English translation. Down the road, there will be lots who will use the book.

Common Problems Treated

A lot of the problems I treat have to do with pills. They're burning your stomach out with pills: antibiotics, Tylenol, sugar diabetes pills; after a while the stomach wants to block up and they're uncomfortable and they end up in the hospital with a sky-high temperature and puffed-up bellies. I think the doctors are pumping them out. It's a new thing but we've been doctoring it for the last ten years or so. To treat that, I boil herbs and make them drink it. After they're cleaned out, if there's any ulcers, they heal. After they heal, many people go back to taking pills again.

I also treat diabetes, heart problems, ear problems, high blood pressure, cuts, toothaches, diarrhea. Also people hear noises, someone talking in their ears—quite a bit of that lately. Another one we do lots is marriage consulting, young people, old people who are ready to break up. We talk to them, pray over them so their marriage will get better. I talk to parents about showing love to their teenagers so there'll be less suicide from the young people. In the case of cancer, I give them medicine if they come out of the hospital and progress is slow. Then they may pop out of it in a hurry. Or if one side doesn't work, I give them herbs to get the other side working again.

You have to realize that nowadays we have a different generation. My generation, sixty to seventy, there are not that many alive, one here and there, so anybody under forty years old is hardly ever introduced to Indian medicine because there are not that many elders to teach them. I treat people mostly between forty and seventy. But they usually don't bring their children because the kids don't know what's going on. They don't even trust traditional things; you can tell by the eyes; you can tell by the body. If an older person brings a daughter and she gets better, she will soon forget all about it. The ones who are teaching culture, they might stay in campsites, but they don't know anything about herbs. They might recognize Rat Root if you show them a plant, but they can't take the kids into the swamp to find Rat Root. Why should they be teaching? They should have an elder who knows something. I also treat curses. There's a lot of that, especially to the east in Saskatchewan. People run to Saskatchewan to get bad medicine to use against people here. It's been going on for the last decade.

Survival of Native Medicine

I am often asked about the relationship between using herbs, psychological counseling, ceremonies, and praying. They are all equally important. You're communicating with the same spirits; they're still God's helpers. The spirits that are running the sun dance in other places, such as the North Wind, South Wind, or Thunder Spirit, they are the same ones we call upon here. So when you go over there to have a dance with them, most of the sun dances are for sick people. Maybe somebody has real bad cancer. Maybe somebody was hurt in a vehicle accident. Others will go because their son doesn't want to stop drinking. So the older ones are up there dancing. But we're slowly losing all those elders. I also hope to pass on how to do ceremonies and counseling to my kids and other young people.

Native medicine will survive but it will have to creep through the cracks. You also must remember that there are some religions that are completely against it, those that started five decades or so ago. And the animals are slowly disappearing, as are the plants and birds. It will be tough. Even if World War III started, how are the people going to survive? They might think they'll be OK, that they'll just live off the plants and animals. They don't realize what will happen.

Hopefully, there will be a revival of Indian medicine in the future. There will be nothing else to use when the bad times come. Doctors have been here in Alberta only a little over a hundred years. The oldest building in Canada is how old? Probably less than five hundred years. That oldest building is not the hospital either. The Indians were doctoring the white people who showed up the first few years. Maybe we will have to go back a step to a time when people were using herbs and trees. People are having a lot of sickness because of the chemicals. If you go into the hospital, you may come out with a different sickness. We don't know the side effects. The old people don't trust them. The younger people don't think until they land in the hospital or jail. The young people don't think ahead. It's scary.

Since the plants are disappearing due to logging and farming, and there are not too many young people interested in learning, and the elders are dying, the most important things that need to be done right away to save traditional medicine are to try to make the oil companies aware of where the plants are, but I'm not there all the time. That's why we need the books bad. We could tell the oil companies that when they see a particular kind of area, such as shown in the book, they should go around it. The oil companies are pretty cooperative. Mind you, we haven't given them very much static because there are so many clear-cuts that almost everything is already gone. If it isn't gone, it will be sprayed anyway, five years down the road. But we will tell them that if there's a natural salt lick to go around, or point out certain herbs that they should avoid. Right now we're going along with them; we're not saying too much. The pipelines are already made. There's no use trying to stop them. What we would like to try to do, if we can find someone to finance it, is to try to transplant plants from a right-of-way to see if they would grow. If someone could move them over to another area that's in the same climate zone, the flowers could grow and the seeds could start flying.

Working with Non-Native Doctors

Native doctors should be trying to work with non-Native doctors, but there are a lot of doctors who don't want anything to do with Native doctors. Do you remember those doctors who volunteered to work with us in the '80s? I think a lot of them have backed away. But they do have interpreters, those who speak Cree, in the hospitals, in various places. They tell the doctors what the patients want.

When people come in with curses, the doctors can't do too much. They have to send the patients back home. This is where the doctors and the traditional Native healers should work together. They should be able to call the healer and take care of it right there. But they're not doing that yet. Once we open that door, it can pop up anywhere.

The Future

Some of the predictions the Natives made in the 1800s have come true. Look at the white buffalo. They had said it would show up in the future. I have a picture right here from when they brought the white buffalo from North Dakota to Calgary. You should have seen the Natives go marching in from all over Canada. We took some of his hair from the fence. That's amazing since they predicted that long ago. There are a lot of predictions that people laugh at, such as that a time will come when money is no good or that trees will be very important. People laugh, thinking it is Indian thought. But I think we're slowly going into it. Not in our time, thank God, but in our children's time. There will be horrible weather because of lack of trees. Heat will hit hard if there's no trees. Millions or billions of trees are being cut every year around the globe. You can't keep that up.

People will try to survive. But they will need a different kind of building that can withstand the winds. They will know, I guess, what to do. As far as the plants are concerned, one of the reasons there is a lot of rain is that Nature is trying to clean the land. I have a letter here concerning where they are going to spray around three hundred acres on my trap line alone. What can you do? All you can do is watch. When we look at our children and grandchildren, they don't know anything about how to survive. If you take them out in the bush and tell them they have to use moss for toilet paper, they scream at the top of their lungs. They want hot water. The ones who run camps for young people set camp where there's electricity, gas, and water. They don't want to have a hard time carrying water or looking for wood. They want portable toilets, the whole bit. If something goes wrong, those kinds of things won't be there. So the survival camps are no good. I know how to survive. I fell in the river in the winter right up to my belly. By the time I got the skidoo out of the river, I was soaked from head to toe. I took off everything since it was soaked, including my lighter. I had about fifteen miles to get to my truck. The spark plugs on the skidoo are on top. When I got it running, I drove a little ways to a Spruce bluff. I put branches together and I used the spark plug from the skidoo to start the fire. I had to rinse my clothes, get as much water out as I could, and try to dry them by the fire. I couldn't dry them but I got them nice and warm and put them back on. Then I took off and made it to the truck. But if I hadn't made it to the truck, I was going to do the same thing again. That's survival. But if that happens to any of these kids, they will be found dead, frozen, even if they get out of the water.

In the future if everything breaks down, we won't have that skidoo either. People won't be in the bush. They will all be in one corner of the recreation center starving, because that's all they know how to do. They can't go in the bush to find food because they would get lost and never come out. There are very few people who know north from south when they are in the bush. It's not in their blood anymore.

Chapter Two

Ecological Issues
Important to Willier

I would like to talk a little about environmental issues since the medicinal plants are rapidly disappearing and I have to travel farther and farther to find them. Unless something is done about the environment, Native medicine may not survive. Also, our traditional way of life is at stake since we depend upon the wild animals and birds for our food.

Clearcut

Even the big animals don't want to walk in clearcut areas. When they clearcut, they take all the trees out. Not long ago, they decided to take roots out as well, so they take in a big machine after the area has been clearcut that pulls out the roots, leaving a big hole. They don't replant. Some holes are chest deep all over the clearcut area. The moose won't walk in there because if they fall in a hole, they have trouble getting out or break a leg. They clearcut in winter and spring. When summer comes, the birds come and the frogs start to move around. Baby birds, mice, and frogs fall into the holes and can't get out. So these species start to disappear—also small rabbits, squirrels, and a few snakes. This is their new idea for the past five years.

I told them, you're making booby traps for everything. When you take all of Alberta into account, that's a lot of animals and birds. They're declining fast. I told Forestry that whoever makes the rules should go look for themselves. They say that if they want a permit, it has to be done this way since it's in the rules. They say they will look into it, and that's the end of the matter. We should get all the birdwatchers to take pictures of dead birds. Maybe that would start a commotion.

We Indians can't get anything going. We see it and tell them but they don't pay any attention. We're called shit stirrers. It's a waste of time. Another issue is that when the government plans to sell or lease unimproved land to farmers or to logging firms, half-mile strips of natural environment, including all types such as forest and wetlands, should be left to crisscross the country. This would not only preserve wild plants but provide shelter for wild animals and birds.

A related issue is road development. New roads open up the wilderness to farming, hunting, and other activities that destroy the wild plants and force Native healers to go further and further to find the herbs they need.

Fish

They build dams on some of the streams that go out of the lakes to keep the lake levels up. When the fish try to come back to the lake, they can't get back in. They try. A jackfish can probably jump six feet high, but he can't clear the dam. I told them, let the people eat the fish that are trapped below the dam. People won't take more than six or seven. They say, no, the whole area is closed. If you catch fish, you will get a big fine. I said, why don't you help them? Throw the fish back in. They say, no, we don't have time for that. They finally got the Department of Water and Environment to come and close the other end of the stream up to raise the water in the stream. About sixty fish jumped into the lake in twenty minutes. A couple lawyers came a week later and saw lots of dead fish being eaten by blue herons and bald eagles. They couldn't make it; they killed themselves trying to jump the dam. They could have made a fish ladder at the side.

Also they should put windmills in the lakes to provide oxygen under the ice in the wintertime—keep one area open when the rest of the lake freezes. I've seen this done in smaller areas such as dugouts where they raise rainbow trout. On a big lake you would need about four big windmills. That would give the fish a chance. Also when they put a seismic line across Whitefish Lake, we think they dynamited. When the ice melted, the shores were white with dead fish. They denied it, but we think they did. When we told that to Forestry and Fish and Game, they claim it was due to lack of oxygen. They covered up for the big oil companies.

Ducks

This spring of 2010, June, we saw a great big smoke in the swamp at Grouard. We went racing over there. The grass was on fire. We asked around what's going on. They said we're training water bombers to put out fires. I said there are millions of bird eggs there right now: ducks, geese, blackbirds, seagulls, blue herons, all kinds of birds. They're just starting to hatch. Some are still in the eggs. They can't escape. They burned the whole area. Now this fall, when we tried to hunt, there were very, very few ducks until they came from the north. They stayed only three days and left. They flew south for the winter, but not many came back because their young had died. Every time we talk about things like that, we are treated as troublemakers.

Moose and Deer

The other thing people wonder about is why so many moose and deer are hit on the road. Hundreds of people are killed or crippled. Twenty-five years ago, authorities said there would be no more shooting from the pavement. You have to be a quarter mile from the pavement. If you can't shoot them, they hang around in the protected areas near the highways. If a farmer leaves some bales in the strips between the roads or in fields near the roads, the deer keep crossing the roads and get killed. The farmers should be told to haul that hay away.

Also, farmers don't let people come on to their property to shoot moose. So the deer and moose multiply. They have to adjust and change. From Swan Hills to Kinuso, there's a big area of bush in there. They should run the skidoos back and forth in there where there are fresh animal tracks. The moose will move back. Fish and Game have lots of time. They can do that. When they see lots of tracks, pull the skidoo out and race it back and forth. Hundreds and hundreds are crippled up from hitting moose and deer.

Plants

Back in the 1980s when we were working together, some of the plants were scarce and I had to go further and further to find them. It is worse now, especially the ones that grow in the wetlands. They drain the wetlands to provide access for oil or logging. Pitcher Plants are one of them that are getting rarer and rarer. They have to reserve a big area for Pitcher Plants, and other areas for other plants. They should not be able to drain these areas or the immediately surrounding areas. All together, we probably take lots, but one individual would take at most two garbage bags. Then they have to be dried. But if there's forty medicine men, they would take eighty bags. They won't overharvest it. But if the wetlands are drained, there won't be many left so the remaining ones will be overharvested.

Fires

They're taking so many trees out before they die due to pine beetles, resulting in loss of habitat. The elk are losing the areas where they hide. They used to take trees in a checkerboard pattern. Now they're taking the in-between areas since the trees will die anyway. In a lot of places they should leave the dead trees standing. That would cause some fire hazard, but if they know how to fight fires, it wouldn't be a problem. When they had the checkerboard pattern, little trees two or three feet high would grow on the clearcuts. If they put the firewall on the clearcut, the little trees there, even if they are seven or eight feet high, they don't have cones yet. The cones burn faster than the wood, and the cones shoot. Instead, they make a firewall right against the tall trees to prevent the fire from getting to the little trees. I told them to make the firewall right through the cones; it will stop because the trees are short.

Fire can jump forty feet off the tops of tall trees. When they put the firewall against the tall trees, the fire seems to stop when it runs out of trees. Then they say the fire is under control. I told them it is not under control, since it will continue to burn underground. It will burn every root. The trees will start falling and domino each other, and the fire will run right across the clearcut area or the road and pick up again on the other side.

I worked for them for forty days north of Slave Lake. I kept telling them what to do and they wouldn't listen. We were getting directions from Edmonton, which is so stupid. The one giving directions should be right there with the fire, not in an office in Edmonton. I said this fire is going to make it to the lake. When the fire appeared to stop, we got orders to take out the big equipment and work the other direction. I told them that as soon as we leave, the big trees will fall and the fire will continue to the lake. Sure enough, it made it right to the lake. When the fire comes, the moose run into the lake and wait like a hippo. When the copter comes with a bucket to get water from the lake, the moose run back into the fire. Why not go to a bigger lake not far away and leave the moose in the water?

If they have a big fire on a hill, the fire and smoke go up the hill. It's hard to make a firewall where the fire is because of the smoke. Why not make the firewall on the other side of the hill? The smoke goes to the top and keeps rising, leaving the other side clear. The fireguard should be about thirty feet wide, all bladed down by the Cats. There's nothing left but dirt. The fire bombers shouldn't drop water right on the fire. If you do that, you move the sparks ahead thirty to forty feet. You should drop it in front of the fire so when the fire reaches there, everything is wet. You can even put it a hundred feet in front. When everything is wet, people can walk in there and put out what fire is left after it is mostly burned out. You'd think they could figure out some of that stuff themselves. I asked them if they were really trying to kill the fire or create jobs for themselves. They didn't reply but they didn't invite me to the next meeting.

If the dead trees were left standing, a fire might start if there's no rain with a lot of lightning. But 85 percent of the fires are caused by people with choppers and Cats. They start fires so the big equipment gets hired so they can pay their bills. We saw a small plane one time flying kind of low. All of a sudden we saw this whirling thing—a diesel rag on fire that they dropped. Then the plane headed back toward High Prairie. We went and killed the fire close to my trap line. By the time we got there on horses, it was big enough that we had trouble getting it out. The rich guys hire somebody to start fires for them. Before you know it, their Cats, big trucks, and heavy equipment are all hired. As far as lightning is concerned, it doesn't do that much damage in northern Alberta. They should have controlled fires in the spring and fall. There are great big trees still standing after two hundred, three hundred, seven hundred years. How come they didn't burn by natural fires? Because the buildup on the forest floor was burned off each year. With pine and pine needles that accumulate on the ground for years, it is very hazardous. Why don't people rake that up around their buildings? It should be clean about three hundred feet from a building. It's the needles that cause trees to burn. The other thing you can do is keep watering your roof. Keep things soaked that can catch fire. The only time it is justified to take in the heavy equipment is when a fire is near a town. If man is not interested in the forests, there is never a big fire there. If man is interested in it, such as in Brazil, all kinds of things can happen. Look at Lesser Slave Lake—No. 2 highway west of the lake. That area was not permitted for housing. It is supposed to be a green zone. About three years ago, there was a nice fire between the two roads. Now you can buy a lot there since the trees are gone. You can't stop that kind of thing, because money is at stake. A lot of fires are started by clear plastic water bottles that people leave in the bush. Once, as an experiment, we held a plastic water bottle so the sun was hitting it near some dry moss. After a couple of minutes, at plus 27 degrees C, the moss began to burn. They should outlaw those plastic bottles. The other thing that could be done is to have a system where the power goes off automatically when the wind gets to a certain speed. When the wind is high, it blows down trees that take out power lines. When these lines hit the ground, they start fires in the dead leaves and underbrush.

Chapter Three

Willier's Favorite Healing Stories

I would like to tell a few of my favorite healing stories as an encouragement to other elders and healers to tell their stories before they die and their stories are lost.

Near-Death Experiences of Patients

MY MOTHER

This is kind of a strange story to a lot of people, I guess. My mom was dying about eleven-thirty at night. I held my mom's hand and said I would come back tomorrow. She was not talking. This was in the High Prairie hospital. My sister was there and a couple of others. I left with a friend, to take him home. We went out of the hospital but had not gone very far when the nurses came running out. They said, "Where's that patient? Where's patient? Tell us where she went." They saw a female figure leave with us and they didn't know where she went, to the bathroom, kitchen area, or outside. Some ran outside to find her. But there was nobody with us. We couldn't see anybody, so we left.

In the meantime, my sister and niece were hollering for the nurses because my mother's heart had stopped. But there was nobody there because they were all looking for that woman they just saw. We drove away. The sisters phoned everybody on the reserve. It takes about fifteen minutes to get to the reserve. We met one of my brothers on the road who stopped us and told us to go back to the hospital because our mom had died. I said I'm not going back. I was there right to the end. If she's gone now, there's no more help from us. She's on her way to heaven or wherever she's going. My brother went on to the hospital.

So I calmed down, had a coffee, and went to bed. About three-thirty in the morning, I thought I was sitting up and I visualized these horses coming, just like I was watching a movie. There were three riders coming full tilt and there was dust behind the horses. And I was in that street, beside the road with this young woman. I looked at her and she looked at me. She said, "I'm going to jump on that middle horse." She seemed to be about nineteen with real long hair. We were on our hands and knees watching. The horses came to a halt. She ran and jumped on the middle horse behind the rider. The horses turned around and raced back the other way. I thought, wow, where did they come from? They were dressed like cowboys. I didn't recognize the horses or riders. I woke up and was sitting on the bed. That's when I looked at my watch.

I never thought too much of it with the funeral coming. I had to get things organized. But two or three weeks later, everybody was trying to find pictures of my mom, so they brought in old pictures to see if I could recognize my mom when she was young. One day we went to an elder's house and were having coffee. She said, you know, I have some pictures from a long time ago—your mom when she was young. So she brought out the pictures. It was exactly the same face as the girl who was kneeling beside me in the vision. I had never seen pictures of my mom that young before. I didn't recognize the young woman I was kneeling with. She probably got a ride with my Dad and his two brothers. But when I saw that picture I realized that was my mom who was there with me. The horses took her to the trail she can go on now. She was the one the nurses saw walking out of the hospital with us.

ALFONSE

Note: Alfonse, whose nickname is Alfoose, is an elder David Young met years ago on the Sucker Creek Reserve. He was helping Russell tan skins. He was about eighty-nine years old then. He was still quite strong. There is an amusing story about Alfonse. He was kicked out of the old folks home when he was around ninety for partying and making too much noise. It was the middle of winter. He moved to the bush at minus 40 degrees C and spent the rest of the winter in a tent. Here, Russell tells about Alfoose's near-death and death experience.

Alfoose was the son-in-law of Moostoos' son. Moostoos was a famous medicine man who signed Treaty 8; Moostoos is my great-grandfather. Alfoose was familiar with Moostoos' medicines. He experienced lots of things connected with traditional medicine and being able to understand it really good. Anyways, when he was in his nineties, he had been good throughout the summer. All of a sudden, his bladder stopped working so they rushed him into the High Prairie hospital. He was in a coma by the time they flew him to Edmonton. They said he probably wouldn't make it. They were pumping him, but his heart stopped. They phoned the family and said his heart had stopped. But they got his heart going again. This went on for three or four days, with his heart stopping and going again. Finally, when his heart stopped, they said he's in his nineties anyway so we can't save him. But his heart started again and he sat up and started pulling things off and throwing them. Well, this is what Alfoose recalled about that period when he was dead.

He recalled that he was in a fog, probably when they were taking him to the hospital. He got on a passenger train and headed west from our area toward the mountains, toward British Columbia. After a while, he had to get off the train and then he had to walk with the spirits. But he could not see the face of the spirit who was in front of him all the time. He tried. He even half ran one time to try to see who the spirit was. Then the spirit half ran as well to stay ahead. So he never did see who it was. Anyway, the spirit brought him to the mountains. But first he said, "there was fresh snow and a lot of animals and tracks. We were walking on the trail. There were coyotes, fishers, martin, rabbits of all kinds, moose. It was beautiful weather. It wasn't cold even though there was snow.

"Finally, we got to a great big tipi where there were some elders. There were four men and two old ladies. I was told I could not go beyond that. So we asked, why? We were told that 'Later on, we have something for you to do.' They said, 'We're having a feast here with offerings to the Great Spirit and we will put food in the fire, tea and bannock. We will smoke the pipe and put tobacco in the fire. We want you to watch real closely how we do everything. That's your job.' So they dragged the wood in, broke the branches, and piled them up for the fire. When evening came, they had the feast. I wanted to go past there; there were lots of everything past there—lots of tipis. I was told that that's where I would go later. They started the feast, they prayed, first they smudged everything, all the meat, all the tea, they prayed all around. Everybody smudged themselves, put food on the fire, prayed more, and they ate. When it was time to smoke, they smoked the pipes, prayed, put more tobacco on the fire, and they closed everything up. They said now I had to go back and show the young people how to do it."

That's when Alfoose sat up in bed and started pulling things off. He said, "There is nothing wrong with me." The doctors were amazed that he had so much energy all of a sudden when his heart was stopping on and off. Well, they sent him home two days later. He lived another five or six years after that. He taught young people. He went around teaching them. He said he accomplished what he was sent back for. He actually slowed down on drinking. When he went back to the hospital again, they didn't take him to Edmonton like the last time. Alfonse said his father-in-law and brother-in-law were there; they had died about thirty years ahead of him. Anyways, Alfonse said that the spirits were here to pick him up. He said, "I don't want to go tonight. They are in a rush but I'm not going with them. I want to go in the morning. I told them already. They left but they will probably come back again." We talked. He told his niece that he had signed his pension check and to make sure everyone eats good at the funeral. He said he wanted to smoke. He said he had been smoking as long as he could remember. He said that when they baptized him, he was taller than the priest. That's when they started keeping track of his age and his birthdays. He must have been around fourteen at the time.

Anyway, his brother-in-law and my grandpa were there. So I lighted a cigarette for him and gave it to him. He said, "That's what I used to do for old people." The nurse was mad at us. She went running out and got the doctor. The doctor came in and gave us static. I said, "Well, he wants to smoke with us for the last time as he's leaving in the morning." The doctor said, "He's not going anywhere!" We said, "Oh yeah, he's leaving. Let him smoke." The doctor turned around and left. Then Alfonse said, "The doctors don't realize. They say I'm full of cancer. It's not cancer. It's just old age." The next morning he was dead. He wasn't scared. He was happy to go with the spirits. Before he left, he said that they're here again and very anxious to get going. When I left to take a nap, I had a call twenty minutes later that he had passed. So Alfoose wasn't worried about it. He was actually happy to go.

This was quite different from another phone call from someone who had joined the priesthood and ended up being a Roman Catholic brother for years and years. Anyway, he worked in big churches or up north. If there were big gatherings, he was there to give a talk. When it came time to die about eighty-two years old, I took my mom there. He was so scared, you couldn't believe it. He was hanging on to both sisters with both hands. For seven days this continued. Scared, scared, scared, no matter how much people would pray. Somebody had to be with him constantly for a whole week. I still don't know why he would be scared. The only thing I could think of he didn't see angels or spirits coming to get him. He wanted nothing to do with Indian stuff. Maybe that is why.

When I talked to him, I said, "Did your mom come yet? Did your grandpa come? Somebody that really loved you? We know for a fact that whoever really loved you will come for you. That's the one who will have the permission to come and get you. If it's your mother, dad, sister, someone who really, really has true love for you, that's the one who will come." Let's say if my sister lost her husband, maybe it will be her husband who will be standing there when it comes time to come. So I asked him if anybody had come for him yet. He said, "No." He was just terrified. We don't know what the Roman Catholic teachings are. Maybe they teach that there's hell there or heaven there. In our theory, we suffer enough here; after we die we're going to heaven. Maybe that made a difference, I don't know. When traditional Indians die, they accept death without fear.

WALLY WILLIER (RELATED TO MY DAD'S SISTER)

There's another story about someone who was about to die. Wally Willier's sons and daughters asked me to come and see what was wrong with the old man. He seemed to be spinning out, losing it. When I went over there and talked to him, he was doing fine, sitting up in a chair like this. He was about eighty-nine years old. He was healthy. He and his wife had their own home. But all the children were there sitting around.

He told them that his mom and dad came to visit him and that they wanted him to go. That's what the son and daughter told me. They said he was losing it because he was seeing spirits. He had a big farm next to a stream. He had horses. He said the spirits landed over there. I asked him what they came in, an airplane or a chopper? He said, "No, it is sitting there right now. It is round and has little windows." He said he went partway to them but then he came back. That's when they thought they were going to lose him. While I was talking to him, he said, "Oh, here they come." There was a window and a door. All the people were sitting there. He turned around and he looked and the door opened, and he introduced me.

In the meantime, all those people who were sitting there ran from the living room. They were scared to get introduced to their grandpa or their grandma. He asked them how come they were so short and young. I said, "While you're talking to them, ask them where they come from." He listened for a while and then he said, "They are coming from the foothills of the mountains straight west from us. All the dead people from around here, all the people around the lake, the colony, Whitefish, Wabasca, they are all over there." I said, "Describe the mountains." He said, "The mountain was huge. So that's in a national park over there, the other side of Fort Nelson." That's amazing. He and Alfonse actually said the same thing though they never saw each other. We don't often have the opportunity to talk to people who nearly died so they could describe the area where they went. They don't see tunnels or light; they see people. He said everybody's happy and that's where the spirits were going to take him for a ride on that spaceship.

So I doctored him then and I told him and all the people who were there, "They all love you and care for you. That's why they're all here. Tell the spirits that you're going to hang on here for another four or five years." So he cried and told the spirits, "I will stay here with my kids." Then he jumped up and said, "Oh, they're leaving; they're leaving. They just flew away." He lived another five years because of the love of his kids. The spirits couldn't pull him away. After that he was back to normal, as if nothing had happened. I am sure that if he had lain down, he would have died since his spirit wanted to go. When he got sick the second time and they phoned me to go doctor him, I said, "No, I'm not" because I remembered what I had said to him—stay around with us for a while. So he passed on.

Predicaments in Which Healers Can Find Themselves

The predicaments described in the following two stories were not funny at the time. In retrospect, however, Russell Willier finds them enormously humorous. His accounts were accompanied at points by roaring laughter, such as when he found himself at a sun dance without enough money to return home, or when he took part in a sweat lodge that was so hot that he didn't know if he would survive.

WE DON'T NEED YOUR MONEY

My friend got ahold of me and said, "There's going to be a sun dance in Spiritwood, Saskatchewan. Come on over." He was working in Saskatchewan at the time, not very far from there. So I said, "OK. When is it?" So he told me when and said to start fasting the Tuesday before that. I said, "OK. I will fast one day, and the next day I will drive." That would make it two days. That was agreeable, so that's what I did. I only had a couple of hundred dollars. I figured that would be enough for gas there and back. I won't need any more anyway since I will be fasting on the way there. So I went racing over there. On the way between St. Paul and Cold Lake, I had two blowouts on the station wagon. So now I had to buy tires. After I bought tires, I didn't have very much money left. I still had enough gas to make it to my friend's place. I told him about my problem of having to buy tires and that I only had about three-quarters of a tank of gas left. We still had to go quite a ways south to go to the sun dance. He said, "We're ready to go but we can't go until we load these cattle to take to the sun dance for people to eat. Can you help us? We'll push them into the corral and load them up." But the corral was no good. The minute we put them in, they came right back out. So we had to fix the corral. Here I was, the second day of not eating and drinking. I was burnt out and I was hot. I was dehydrated. This was in August. Finally I told him, "Why not shoot the cattle and bring the meat in? It would be a lot easier." "No," he said. "They want the cattle alive." Finally we got the cattle loaded and made it to the sun dance.

When we got in, the cows were still in the trailer. They didn't get out until the next day. We had to camp out. We camped in a vacant house with lights on, and nobody really slept good. We had to be up at five in the morning to go get the tree. I figured, well, since I'm burnt out I'll go help get the tree. When the tree gets here, I'll sneak out and go sleep in my station wagon until they're done around three in the afternoon. I had it all figured out. We were out there cutting the tree, bringing it down, bringing it to the circle, slowly. We would stop and pray, three or four times. It was a big poplar tree, probably fourteen inches in diameter. Most of the branches were left on. Now they wanted somebody to sit there and watch the tree and smudge it on and off until the old man directing the sun dance got there. Everybody wanted to leave. They said to me, "Why don't you stay here. You've got no kids. You came alone. You can do it until the old man gets here, maybe about ten." It was about six-thirty. I had no choice but to stay there. Then it started raining. It poured and poured all day.

At around two, the old man finally showed up. The others were busy. Nobody came to meet him. They were chopping willows and little poplars and making the whole thing. The big tree was going to come in next. The old man knew I was very tired. I was soaked head to toes. There was no shelter. My cowboy hat was the only thing that kept the fungus dry. The rest of the funguses were in a plastic bag. They were still moist and hard to light. The old man was ninety-seven years old. He came limping in. I thought that he was the elder in charge of the sun dance. I talked to him for a while. He said, "I'm not in charge. The one in charge is my dad; he should be coming in soon." Finally the old man came in a van. They took him out and he was in a wheelchair. He got out and came over to where I was. I got introduced to him. He started talking and he said, "You must be pretty tired. You don't even have a shirt on." I said, "It is soaked anyway."

He talked to his son and said, "How many times have I told you guys to get some tobacco and pray so the rain will stop?" Somebody went and got tobacco and gave it to him. You could see that the clouds broke up where the sun dance was. It was raining about two hundred yards away but nothing at the sun dance site. Nothing after that for three or four days. It was kind of misty but not raining. This old man was 116 years old. He said this was his last year. He was going to pass it all on to his great-great-great-grandson who was twenty-two years old. So we talked and talked. He said, "There was a great, powerful medicine man over there west end of Lesser Slave Lake. He's known as Moostoos. Is he any relation to you?" I was surprised. I said, "Yeah, he's my great-grandpa." He told me that his dad and grandpa knew Moostoos, who died around 1917. Anyway, he said, "You must be tired. I don't want you to hallucinate. You're going to be seeing spirits tomorrow or the day after. What I want you to do tonight when we're done here, when the sun goes down, go eat as much as you can and drink as much as you can, and sleep. When morning comes, if you get up before sunup, eat some more. Drink lots of water, be ready. You already fasted enough. You've already tortured yourself by chasing cows." He knew that even though I hadn't told him. He told me a lot of things I never told him. I was pretty surprised.

The tree was put up, and the singing started right away. I danced that evening. That night I went and had a real good sleep in my car. The next day we were dancing all day and I saw some spirits. They were powerful ones. There were probably five hundred or six hundred people there by that time. There's a big circle of cars, vehicles, and tents around the tree. The ones further inside are the ones who were fasting and dancing, but they could smell the bacon! They could smell the meat being cooked in the frying pan. On one side were all women and girls; on the other side were men. In the central area, to the north, were the drummers and singers. The elders were walking around the tree. They would pick up a print and pray for an individual to be healed. There were a lot of people watching. Lots of people came to be prayed over by the elders and to ask for help with a certain problem. I saw eight spirits at the dance. I saw the Grandmother Willow, the old lady; the Thunder Spirit, a very important one. He was just as tall as the sun dance tree, at least forty feet, and his hair was all colored, every color you could imagine; that's how I knew he was the Thunder Spirit, as he had been described to me before.

Half of his shirt was white and the other half was red. You could just see the muscles—something like Mr. Clean but as tall as the trees. He was looking at all the old ladies, taking his time looking at them. Then he looked at the drummers. Then he started looking at the men on that side. Then all of a sudden he saw me. His eyes fixed and stopped on me. Most people didn't seem to see him. He looked at me for about three minutes. He was standing right against the tree in the middle of the lodge. There were songs so I kept dancing. I asked him if he would be there to help me when I doctored people. He rolled his head and then disappeared. I also saw the Buffalo Spirit and a white moose, a young calf moose, the different winds representing the four directions. There were hundreds of prints hanging on the tree, all over the branches and also on the main stem. What you're told to do is pray while facing the tree at all times. Don't be looking around all over. Concentrate on one spirit while you're praying and dancing. That's the information they gave us. There was no wind or rain, but one of the prints started shaking.

Then all of a sudden, a blue-looking man showed up, the West Wind. Medicine people were doctoring there, but I didn't see any spirit go to help. The medicine people were praying and holding prints around the bottom of the tree. You have to ignore all that commotion and concentrate on the tree, so I didn't notice if the spirits helped with the healing. There was a lot of drumming for the dancers. Everybody had eagle bone whistles, so it was noisy. If you don't concentrate the way you are supposed to, the spirits will bypass you and not look at you. So a lot of people don't see the spirits. It was a real struggle for me all the way.

I was watching all these people putting money in a big tub: $20 bills, $10 bills that were going to be given to those who had come from a long ways. They don't count the money. They just grab a handful and give it to those who need it on the last day. People went up and said where they were from and they were given money. Finally, it was my turn. I was banking on this to get home since I had no cash left. My friend waved at me to come over, so I went over there. I was standing there and he made a speech. He said, "Oh no, we don't need your money. All we wanted was your prayers. Thank you for everything." I was stunned because I never got a dollar from that tub! This was the fourth day. The sun dance itself takes two days: one day to put up the tree and one day of dancing.

I had half a tank of gas. I was stuck in the middle of Saskatchewan with a long ways to go home. I'm beat and tired. So I had a surprise when people started coming to the station wagon and asked if they could get help. I asked them, "Who sent you?" They said, "The old man who was running the sun dance; he sent us to you." I was surprised. I guess he knew what kind of problems I could help with. So I had five there to doctor. Since I didn't get any money at the sun dance, now I had to try to earn it. They gave me gifts when I doctored them. To make the story short, they gave me slippers, a small vest that didn't fit, and a horse. I was pouring sweat now wondering if someone was even going to give me $20 so I could get back to Alberta. Since my friend lives there, I gave the horse to him to keep for me until I could pick it up a year later. It was pretty old when I got it. It didn't do me much good. If he had given me $30 I would have been happy.

Finally one gave me $20 and another gave me two $20 bills. I stayed for a week doctoring people. My friend said, "This is a lesson for you to take more money with you." I said, "How can it be a lesson? When you're broke, you're broke. If I had had more money, I would have carried more money. We never have any money anyway." I told that story to the people in Sucker Creek. They said I should have killed him. They thought it was one of the funniest stories they had ever heard.

THE SWEAT LODGE

I'll tell you another good story. We were at another sun dance in Duffield, Alberta. Harold Cardinal asked me to go with him. He said, "I always go to that sun dance over there." I said, "OK." I didn't really want to go along, but I was doctoring Harold at that time. He was really sick before, but now he was starting to move around so he asked me to go with him. I didn't want to turn him down so I went. I said, "I'm not dancing; I'll stay in the tent area with your wife and my missus" (which was Yvonne then). He said, "OK. No problem." I planned to watch. I didn't fast or anything. I just sat back and relaxed.

They had the sweat lodge going now. They were hollering and walking around. They needed people to go in the sweat lodge to open the sun dance. I never budged. All of a sudden I saw somebody coming. I knew what was going to happen. Harold was walking toward me. I said, "What's wrong?" He said, "We're short one human for the sweat. We have to represent north, south, east, west." He had three with him, plus the guy who sings and the guy who pours water on the hot coals. He said, "Can you come and help us? We're stuck because nobody wants to go." So I said, "I guess." I just wanted to relax and see how they do things over here. Now I'm dragged into representing one of the four directions in a sweat.

I got in my shorts and my towel. The sweat lodge was kind of small. In the middle, the rocks were on top of the ground rather than being in a pit. I had to crawl around the rocks and sit on the other side. We were sitting really close to the rocks, about two feet away at the most. The rocks were all red, and they closed the door. The medicine man started singing. I was representing the south and sitting on the south. It was hot! Really hot and burning my ears. My friend Harold was hollering and screaming it was so hot. I figured, oh gosh. Am I going to make it? I prayed for a while but then I couldn't pray; it was just too hot. I wasn't going to move. I figured I would just stiffen up and take the heat. I figured they would open the door pretty soon, but they never opened the door. They stopped singing after four real long songs, probably four or five minutes per song, instead of the more normal two minutes. When they finished singing, you could see the rocks hissing and anytime they poured water, the steam was thick.

Now I knew why nobody wanted to go to that sweat lodge. But now it was too late. I asked myself, what kind of friends have I got, dragging me into this thing. They said, the door will not open until we're done. I knew I had to stay there another three rounds. Each round was fifteen minutes. The door was not opened between rounds. When you have a pit for the rocks, it's not so bad; when you pour water into the pit, the steam goes upward; here when they poured the water on the rocks, the steam went sideways. It was getting Harold right on the legs. He was raw. He was moaning and groaning. He couldn't do anything. I would have moved out of that spot but there wasn't enough room to move anywhere, even a foot. He said he had his big towel in front of him but the steam still went right through. Was I ever glad when that was over. I went back. I said to Harold, "What kind of friend are you?" After that, we went to Edmonton and then home. I was going to go hunting. I asked Harold if he wanted to go hunting with me. He said, "No, that's OK." So I decided to go by myself. I drove a little ways, pulled over, and slept in the truck. At five in the morning, before daybreak, I heard the eagle whistle and the rattle, what I had heard for three days at the sun dance. The spirits woke me up. So I got up and smudged the rifle and drove just a couple of hundred yards. There were two big moose right on the road, walking right toward me. If the spirits hadn't woke me up, I would have missed them. As it was, I got them both. Since they were right on the road, all I had to do was skin them, throw them in the truck, and go home.

Another time after a sun dance at the Alexander Reserve, we were driving home. We looked up a cut line and saw an elk standing there. I said, we might as well take it. So I stopped and shot him and took him home. It was easy to get. It wasn't cagey. A lot of times when you go hunting, the animals are real cagey; they're running already and you don't see them again. Going to something like a sun dance makes a big difference.

Part II

Russell Willier's Medicine Bundle

Part II consists of two chapters. Chapter Four describes a field trip in 2011 when David Young traveled more than 1,000 kilometers with Russell Willier to find plants used in his healing practice. Chapter Five describes each plant in Willier's medicine bundle, illustrated with photographs of what a plant looks like in the summer and in the fall. Photographs are by David Young, unless otherwise noted. Robert Rogers, coauthor of the book, has provided additional information for each plant, to supplement the information provided by Russell Willier.

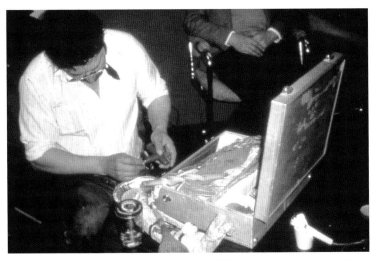

Russell Willier's modern "medicine bundle" containing herbs, animal and bird parts, minerals, and ritual objects such as a pipe and rattle

Chapter Four

Field Trip, Summer 2011

David Young visited Russell Willier in July 2011 so they could travel to the different areas where Willier picks his medicinal herbs. The purpose of this field trip was to photograph the plants when they were in full bloom or bearing fruit. Because Willier believes it is important to document the kinds of environments in which plants are growing, Young took several general photographs whenever they stopped, followed by close-up photographs of individual plants. If there was some doubt about the identity of the plant, they took samples of the entire plant, including roots, and enclosed the plant between sheets of heavy white paper, sealed with tape. Willier's name for the plant was written on the outside of each packet. The purpose of preserving plants in this way was to assist Robert Rogers, a botanist and coauthor of this book, to provide a positive identification.

Young visited Willier again in October 2011 to photograph the same plants as they appear after the frost and are ready to be harvested. This second trip followed the same route as the first. They also visited a couple of additional places to photograph plants they had not been able to find on the first trip. On the first trip, Willier and Young were assisted by Willier's son, Russell Jr., and later on by Willier's partner, Norma. On the second trip they were assisted for the entire trip by Russell Jr. and Norma. On the first trip, they traveled more than 1,000 kilometers and made thirteen stops to photograph plants. The descriptions of these stops in the following pages are taken directly from Young's research diary for the July trip. Because they followed the same route for the October trip, that trip is not described.

Unless indicated otherwise, all photographs are by David Young. Those marked "research team" were taken by individuals on the 1985 field trips; photographs contributed by Robert Rogers are so indicated.

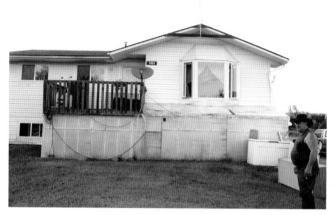

Russell Willier's house on the Sucker Creek Reserve,
northern Alberta

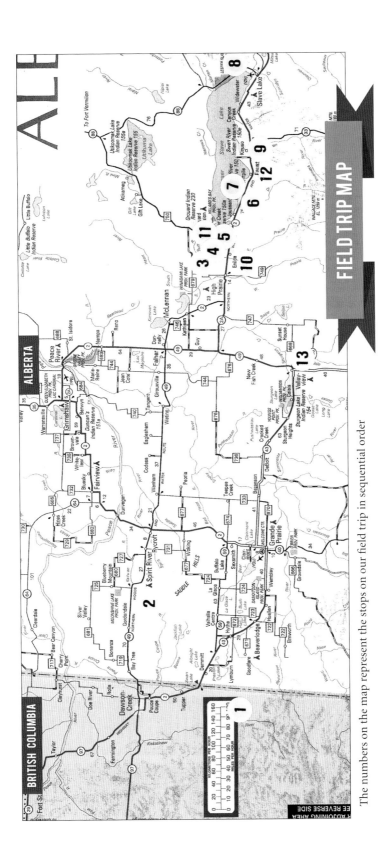

The numbers on the map represent the stops on our field trip in sequential order

Stop 1

Traveling from Vancouver Island, I arrived by plane in Grande Prairie, Alberta, at four in the afternoon on July 12, 2011. Russell Willier and his son, Russell Jr., picked me up in a fifteen-year-old truck. I loaded my bags in the open back that was already full of camping equipment. The front was a little crowded too for three people. We drove to a spot near Kelly Lake, British Columbia, where we photographed Northern Valerian (*Valeriana dioica*), Purple Avens (*Geum rivale*), Diamond Willow (*Salix bebbiana*), Tamarack (*Larix laricina*), Jack Pine (*Pinus banksiana*), Indian Paintbrush (*Castilleja raupii*), Red Osier Dogwood (*Cornus stolonifera*), Lungwort (*Mertensia paniculata*), Black Spruce (*Picea mariana*), and Wild Aster (*Aster puniceus*).

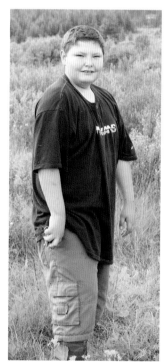
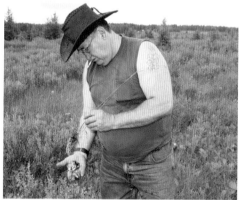
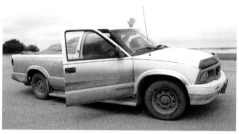

Clockwise from left: Russell Jr.; Russell; Our truck

STOP 1 HABITAT

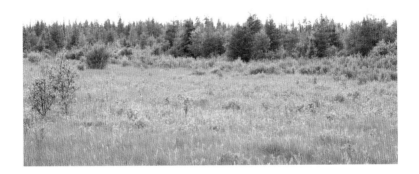

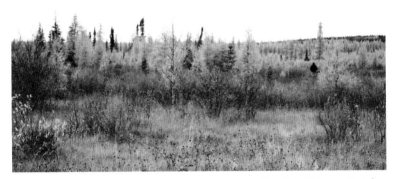

Top: July; Bottom: October

Stop 2

We then drove to Dawson Creek, British Columbia, where we stopped for lunch. After eating, we crossed back into Alberta and drove north to a spot about thirty-five miles south of Spirit River, where we took a dirt road into the bush to a camping spot in a swampy area Russell has used before. We camped between two signs that said "Absolutely No Camping!" It was about 10:00 p.m. by the time we got the tent set up and the air mattresses inflated.

I was exhausted, so I crawled into bed while Russell and his son took off down the dirt road with a gun to look for moose. I did not hear them return, without a moose. When I arose at about two in the morning to go to the toilet, I didn't need a flashlight because it doesn't get very dark this far north at this time of year. We all slept in until eight the next morning (July 13) and then got up to fix coffee and fry some ham over an old camp stove.

After breakfast, I took some photos of plants in the immediate area: Wild Mint (*Mentha arvensis*), Wild Rose (*Rosa woodsii*), Angelica (*Angelica genuflexa*), Cow Parsnip (*Heracleum lanatum*), Diamond Willow (*Salix bebbiana*), Diamond Willow Fungus (*Haploporus odorus*), Green Alder (*Alnus crispa*), Wild Sarsaparilla (*Aralia nudicaulis*), and Labrador Tea (*Ledum groenlandicum*). We then hopped in the truck and drove up the mud road to a well-trampled area where moose come to lick the deposits that a salt spring brings out of the ground. We came across a young bear there. We took some photos in the area and then continued up the road as far as we could in search of Balsam Fir (*Abies balsamea*), but were forced to turn around as the road became impassable. On the way back, we stopped to photograph False Solomon's Seal (*Smilacina racemosa*), Fireweed (*Epilobium angustifolium*), and Trembling Aspen (*Populus tremuloides*). After returning to camp, I walked up the road a fair distance to find a place to do my morning business. I found a downed tree to sit on and unwittingly settled into a nest of Stinging Nettle. The experience stayed with me the rest of the morning.

STOP 2 HABITAT

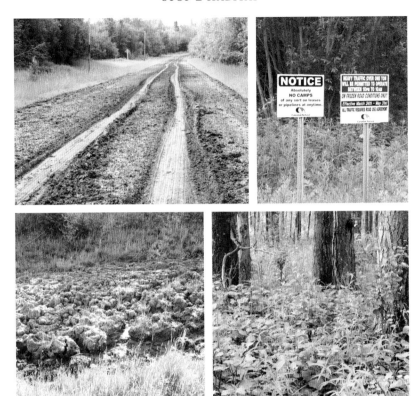

Clockwise from top left: Mud road; Swampy area where we camped;
Habitat for False Solomon's Seal; Salt lick

Stop 3

After packing up camp, we traveled to Spirit River, where we picked
up Route 49 east, passing vast fields of peas, canola, timothy grass, and
wheat. We stopped in Rycroft for lunch, after which we continued to
McLennan. A little later we stopped at the Big Prairie community hall
to photograph Gumweed (*Grindelia squarrosa*), Sage (*Artemisia frigida*), and Canadian Goldenrod (*Solidago canadensis*).

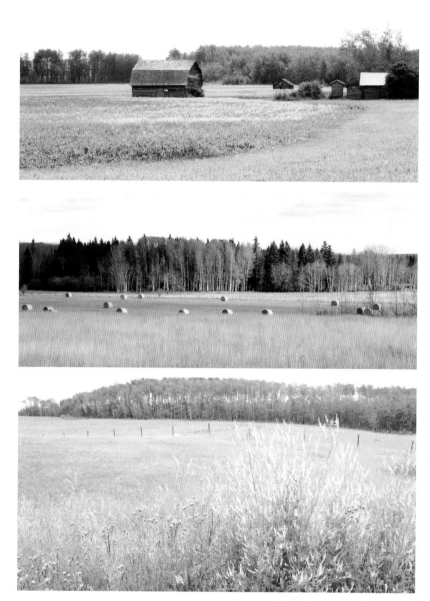

Top to bottom: July; October;
Field behind the Big Prairie community hall in July

Stop 4

We then took a dirt road toward Grouard, stopping to photograph Balsam Fir (*Abies balsamea*) and White Spruce (*Picea glauca*).

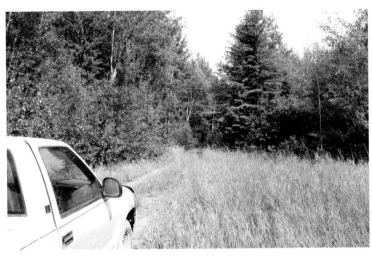

July

Stop 5

Our final stop before reaching home was Grouard, where we filled up with gas and then drove on to the Sucker Creek Reserve, arriving around 9:00 p.m., having traveled around 700 kilometers to find our plants. By the end of the day, we had photographed around 90 percent of Russell's repertoire. We were way ahead of schedule because of the good weather and because Russell knows exactly where to go for each kind of plant. After supper, we went to a swampy area near the railroad track on the Sucker Creek Reserve to photograph Saskatoon Berry (*Amelanchier alnifolia*), Purple-stemmed Aster (*Aster puniceus*), Seneca Snake Root (*Polygala senega*), Yellow Pond Lily (*Nuphar variegatum*), Red Clover (*Trifolium pratense*), and Stinging Nettle (*Urtica dioica*).

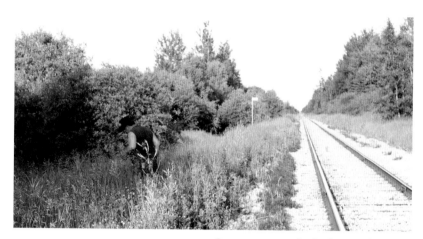

Swampy area on the Sucker Creek Reserve

Stop 6

The next day (July 14), I spent the morning identifying and labeling the photographs we had taken so far. I made a sandwich for lunch, after which Russell, Norma, and I drove toward Lesser Slave Lake, stopping along the road to photograph Narrow Spinulose Shield Fern (*Dryopteris carthusiana*).

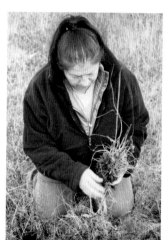 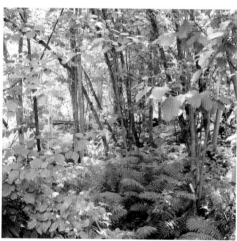

Left: Norma; Right: Habitat for Narrow Spinulose Shield Fern

Stop 7

About halfway to Lesser Slave Lake, we turned north for a few miles, where we stopped to photograph Sweet Flag (*Acorus americanus*) in a swampy area just inside the fence of a farmer's field.

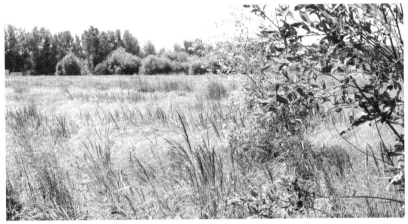

Sweet Flag habitat

Stop 8

We then continued on to Lesser Slave Lake, recently burned out by a fire. We went through what was left of the town and partway around the lake, traveling north. Then we turned right on a gravel road and went as far as we could until the road was flooded with water. Norma stayed in the truck while Russell and I walked about three miles to where we could wade into the swamp along the road to find Pitcher Plant (*Sarracenia purpurea*). We photographed a couple of Pitcher Plants, Peat Moss (*Sphagnum fuscum*), and Waxpaper Lichen (*Parmelia sulcata*) and then started back, stopping to photograph Paper Birch (*Betula papyrifera*), Bog Birch (*Betula pumila* or *B. nana*), Wild Strawberry (*Fragaria virginiana*), Raspberry (*Rubus idaeus* or *R. strigosus*), Buffalo Berry (*Shepherdia canadensis*), Cattail (*Typha latifolia*), Northern Gooseberry (*Ribes oxyacanthoides*), Wild Rose (*Rosa woodsii*), and Arctic Raspberry (*Rubus arcticus*). We returned to the truck and traveled a little further north to a park, where we photographed Creeping

Wintergreen (*Gaultheria hispidula*), after which we returned to Lesser Slave Lake, where we ate supper and visited the hospital where Russell had promised to visit the friend of one of his nieces. By the time we arrived there, the friend had already gone home.

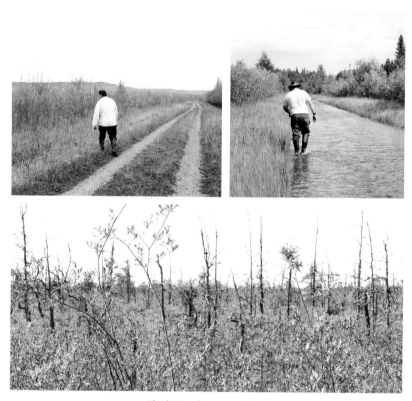

Clockwise from top left: October; Flooded road in July;
Pitcher Plant habitat

Stop 9

We then went on to Kinuso, where we parked the truck and Russell and I hiked along a dike protecting the town to where we could photograph some of the main plants used in a combination to break bad curses: High Bush Cranberry (*Viburnum opulus*), Choke Cherry (*Prunus virginiana*), Pin Cherry (*Prunus pensylvanica*), and Hazelnut (*Corylus cornuta*). We photographed Black Poplar (*Populus balsamifera*) on the way home. When we arrived home, we packaged some of the plants we had collected. I went to bed around ten. The next morning (July 15), we got up at nine and had breakfast. I then interviewed Russell about some of the plants that I had photographed but about which I had no information. Russell informed me that the most basic plants in his medicine bundle are Sweet Flag (*Acorus americanus*), Purple-stemmed Aster (*Aster puniceus*), Northern Valerian (*Valeriana dioica*), Yellow Pond Lily (*Nuphar variegatum*), and Seneca Snake Root (*Polygala senega*). He said that if you have these plants, you can deal with just about anything. About twelve-thirty, Russell went to town to buy dog food, and I took one of Russell's two quads out for a practice ride along the fence line, turning right onto a cut line to a large field owned by Russell. I had no trouble with the quad, though I thought I might get stuck a couple of times in large, deep puddles where the wheels spun quite a bit before I got through. I returned home around one. In the afternoon I worked on my notes and packaging some of the plants we had collected earlier. The next morning (July 16), I continued working on organizing the plant photos and attaching scientific names.

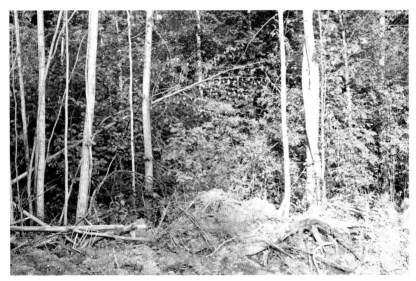

Habitat near Kinuso

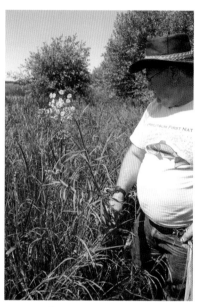

Russell with Spotted Water Hemlock

Stop 10

Later in the morning, Russell and I took the truck on a two-hour round-trip southwest of the reserve toward Enilda Tower to photograph and collect specimens of Spotted Water Hemlock (*Cicuta maculata*).

Stop 11

Around four-thirty, Russell, his son, his granddaughter, and I took two quads on a trip into the fields and bush near Russell's house, driving on otherwise impassable bush roads with some of the puddles deep enough to come up over the running boards. We stopped at one place to pick Sweet Grass (*Hierochloe odorata* [*Anthoxanthum nitens*]), as well as Yellow Avens (*Geum aleppicum* or *G. macrophyllum*), Yarrow (*Achillea millefolium*), Arrow-leaved Coltsfoot (*Petasites sagittatus*), and Twining Honeysuckle (*Lonicera dioica*). We came to a halt at a lake where Russell has a 340-acre hay field. There were hundreds of ducks and geese on the lake where Russell goes for hunting. An African man and his wife from Edmonton were supposed to visit here today, but there was some kind of mix-up. The Edmonton couple thought Russell was coming to Edmonton instead. The wife went to her home country in Africa recently and returned with the mind of a twelve-year-old, apparently due to some kind of dementia. Russell thinks she was cursed while in Africa. The next morning (July 17), I interviewed Russell about general issues such as how he became a medicine man, the current state of Indian medicine, etc. Among many other things, Russell said that when someone gives him a new combination or trades one with him, he will not use it until after he has observed its effects on a patient of the healer who gave him the combination.

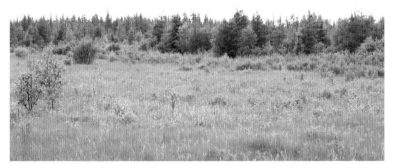

Fields and bush near Russell's home

Stop 12

After lunch we stopped on the reserve to photograph American Mountain Ash (*Sorbus americana* or *S. decora*), and then went to Faust to visit Albert and Emmy New. Albert is an eighty-seven-year-old medicine man who has exchanged combinations with Russell. Albert has an herb shack where he has jars of labeled, dried herbs, as well as herbs hanging from the ceiling. The shack is heated with a wood stove. Russell took a combination, including Arbutus (*Arbutus menziesii*) from British Columbia, for Emmy because she is having trouble walking after several bypass surgeries in which arteries were taken from her legs. Though Arbutus is not part of Russell's traditional repertoire, he was impressed while visiting our home on Gabriola Island that an Arbutus tree will heal over a wound pretty quickly with new growth. He intends to experiment with it on some patients in Alberta. After Russell doctored Emmy, we were invited into the house (an old but very neat and cozy trailer), where we were served bannock and tea. We returned home about two-thirty in the afternoon, at which time I brought these field notes up to date. The next morning (July 18), I went over all of the data to ensure that it is complete. I also reviewed all of the Cree names for the plants, trying to spell them phonetically so they can be pronounced in a way that is similar to the way Russell says them. This afternoon, Russell got out his tipi cover to examine. It is in good shape, so Russell gave it to me to pay me back for money I loaned him some years earlier. Emmy New called to say that she was already getting better from the treatment.

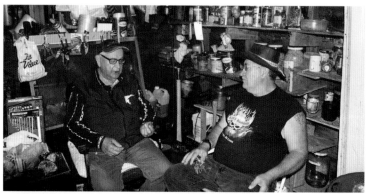

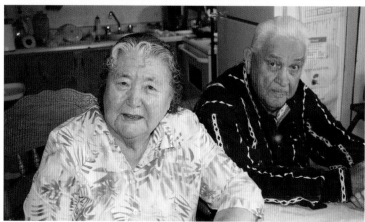

Top: Albert and Russell talking in Albert's shack;
Bottom: Albert and Emmy New

Stop 13

The next morning (July 19), we left early for Grande Prairie, stopping near Valleyview to photograph and pick Buffalo Berry (*Shepherdia canadensis*) and Wolf Willow (*Elaeagnus commutata*). We also took photographs of Dandelion (*Taraxacum officinale*) and Purple Vetch

(*Vicia cracca*). I left by plane to return home around one-thirty in the afternoon, having achieved all we had hoped to do on the research trip. Russell has people coming from Goodfish Lake and Edmonton on Thursday and Saturday for doctoring. Otherwise, he would go moose hunting. Russell seems to have two or three parties a week come for doctoring. He sometimes goes to other places to doctor or for counseling. Not too long ago, he was asked to go to Fox Lake, an isolated community in the north, to counsel young people who were sniffing gasoline. Some of these young people had never been out of their community to cross the Peace River by ferry as it is too expensive. Russell helped run a survival camp for the community, but he says such camps are a waste of time as they want all the luxuries such as toilets and electricity. He says that most young people would not be able to survive if they were stranded in the bush or if the services went down. Sometime during the day, Russell mentioned that the combination he had prepared for my wife, Michiko, when she was in a coma in 1987, consisted of plants for removing a curse, plus Green Alder (*Alnus crispa*). He also told me that the four plants for opening the door to the spiritual world are Sweet Grass (*Hierochloe odorata*) and Diamond Willow Fungus (*Haploporus odorus*), used in Alberta; Sage (*Artemisia frigida*), used in the prairies; and Western Red Cedar (*Thuja plicata*), used in the West.

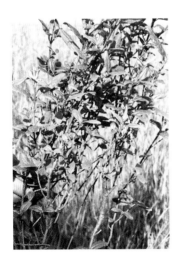 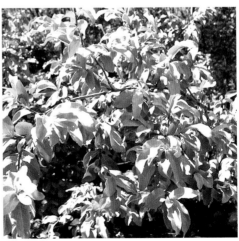

Left: Buffalo Berry; Right: Wolf Willow

Chapter Five

Plants Used by Russell Willier

Plants in Willier's Medicine Bundle

Scientific Name
Common English Name
Cree Name Used by Willier
English Name Used by Willier

———————

Abies balsamea
Balsam Fir
napakâsîta
Flat-needle Spruce

Achillea millefolium
Yarrow
wapanowask
Morning Flower

Acorus americanus
Calamus, Sweet Flag, Flagroot
wiyikiyo
Rat Root

Alnus crispa
Green Alder
atôspi
Hill Willow

Amelanchier alnifolia
Saskatoon
saskahtômina
Saskatoon Berry

Angelica genuflexa
Angelica
wacaskowîykomawask
Rat Smell Root

Aralia nudicaulis
Wild Sarsaparilla
waposociyipîyk
Bear Root

Arbutus menziesii
Arbutus, Madrona, Pacific Madrone
*None, as this is an import from
the West Coast of Canada.*
Arbutus

Artemisia frigida
Sage, Sagebrush, Prairie
Sagewort, Pasture Sage
mostoswiyikwaskwa
Buffalo Grass

Aster puniceus
Purple-stemmed Aster, Wild
Aster, Aster, Wild Blue Aster
*misiyistakîyowask, iskomaski-
yikêy*
Big Arrow, Morning Flower

Betula papyrifera
Paper Birch, White Birch
waskwiyî
Birch

Betula pumila or *B. nana*
Bog Birch, Dwarf Birch,
Swamp Birch
apistiwaskwayi
Small Birch

Castilleja raupii
Indian Paintbrush
or Red Paintbrush
okimawask
King Root

Cicuta maculata
Spotted Water Hemlock,
Cowbane
manitoskâtâsk
God's Carrot

Cornus stolonifera
Red Osier Dogwood
mikwapimakwa
Red Willow

Corylus cornuta
Hazelnut
pakanâhtihk
Peanut Willow

Dryopteris carthusiana
Narrow Spinulose Shield Fern
wiyinohwask
Fat Root

Elaeagnus commutata
Wolf Willow
soniyawniyipsi
Silver Willow

Epilobium angustifolium
(*Chamerion angustifolium*)
Fireweed
eskohtiyowaskwa, skohtiyôciyipihk
Fireweed

Fragaria virginiana
Wild Strawberry
ohtihmina
Heart Berry

Gaultheria hispidula
Creeping Wintergreen
apstepakosa
Tiny Leaves

Geum aleppicum or
G. macrophyllum
Yellow Avens, Large-leaved
Yellow Avens
sakohtowask
Love Root, Jealousy Root

Geum rivale
Purple Avens, Water Avens
kiniyipikominanatihk
Snake Root

Grindelia squarrosa
Gumweed
kapikiyowapakwani
Gum Flower

Haploporus odorus
Diamond Willow Fungus
wikiyimakasikan
Diamond Willow Fungus

Heracleum lanatum
Cow Parsnip
pakwânâhtik
Empty Stalk

Hierochloe odorata
(*Anthoxanthum nitens*)
Sweet Grass
wêkaskwa
Sweet Grass

Larix laricina
Tamarack
wakanakahn
Bendable Stem

Ledum groenlandicum (*Rhodo-
dendrom groenlandicum*)
Labrador Tea
maskihkohpakwa
Muskeg Tea

Lonicera dioica
Twining Honeysuckle
payipotakask
Vine with a Hole in the Center

Mentha canadensis or *M.
arvensis ssp. borealis*
Wild Mint
amiskowiyikaskwa
Mint, Beaver Ears Leaves,
Beaver Roots

Mertensia paniculata
Lungwort, Tall Bluebells
kasasiyoyakansiyohk
King's Plant

Nuphar variegatum
Yellow Pond Lily
waskwatamoh
Water Lily

Parmelia sulcata
Waxpaper Lichen
waskwiya
Moss

Petasites sagittatus
Arrow-leaved Coltsfoot
miyokatayinipiya
Frog Leaves

Picea glauca
White Spruce
siyihtah
White Spruce

Picea mariana
Black Spruce
minahyik
Black Spruce

Pinus banksiana
Jack Pine
askatikos
Jack Pine

Polygala senega
Seneca Snake Root, Milkwort,
Seneca Root
miyinsiyikîysa
Bead Berry

Populus balsamifera
Black Poplar, Balsam Poplar
mayîmiyitos
Black Poplar

Populus tremuloides
Trembling Aspen, Aspen Poplar
miyotohs
White Poplar

Prunus pensylvanica
Pin Cherry
nipinimina
Summer Berry
(Summer Willow)

Prunus virginiana
Choke Cherry, Circle Berry
tokwayîminana
Choke Cherry or Circle Berry

Ribes oxyacanthoides
Northern Gooseberry
sapominahk
See-through Berry

Rosa woodsii
Wild Rose
okiniyi
Wild Rose

Rubus arcticus
Arctic Raspberry,
Dwarf Raspberry
oskisikomina
Eye Berry

Rubus idaeus or *R. strigosus*
Raspberry
ayiskanahk
Raspberry

Salix bebbiana
Diamond Willow
nêpisiyiwaskwôto
Diamond Willow

Sarracenia purpurea
Pitcher Plant
ayikitas
Frog Pants

Shepherdia canadensis
Buffalo Berry, Soapberry
kinipiknipsi
Snake Willow

Smilacina racemosa
(*Maianthemum racemosum*)
False Solomon's Seal
kawawkanaht
Backbone Root

Solidago canadensis
Canadian Goldenrod
ohsawicêyipêyihk
Goldenrod

Sorbus americana or *S. decora*
American Mountain Ash
asiniyociyipiyk
Mountain Ash

Sphagnum fuscum
Peat Moss,
Sphagnum Peat Moss
maskwoskwa
Peat Moss

Taraxacum officinale
Dandelion
osawciyipiykwa
Dandelion

Trifolium pratense
Red Clover
mostosmetisowihn
Clover

Typha latifolia
Cattail
ohtawaskwa
Ocean Plant

Urtica dioica
Stinging Nettle
masan
Thistle

Valeriana dioica
Northern Valerian, Marsh
Valerian
apiscakowaskos
Small Arrow

Viburnum opulus (*V. opulus var. americanum*)
High Bush Cranberry, Cramp
Bark
nêpiminana
High Bush Cranberry

Vicia cracca
Purple Vetch, Tufted Vetch
kiyiminkiyowask
Climbing Vine

Total: 61 plants

The orthography of the Cree terms for the plants in Russell Willier's medicine bundle was provided by Clifford Cardinal, a healer, researcher, and professor associated with the Centre for the Cross-Cultural Study of Health and Healing at the University of Alberta. There is, however, substantial variation in the terms used by different Cree healers. The above list of plants in Russell Willier's medicine bundle does not include plants he uses infrequently, such as Sweet Pine, or plants that he obtains from Native groups in southern Alberta. It also does not include a plant we collected on the field trip that we cannot identify. Russell calls it Burnt Willow; it may be a type of wild cherry, such as Black Cherry. Several of the plants depicted in this chapter are described as a "tobacco substitute." This means that they can be used in a pipe for ceremonial purposes. Each plant is associated with the number of the stop where it was photographed. This enables the reader to refer to Chapter Four, where habitat photographs are included for each plant.

The data in the following pages concerning Additional Cree Information, Folk Uses, and Properties have been supplied by Robert Rogers, RH (AHG), coauthor of this book. Rogers also provided the scientific names of the plants presented in the following pages. Rogers is a well-known ethnobotanist with a number of publications on medicinal plants. He is an assistant clinical professor in the Department of Family Medicine at the University of Alberta. Much of the information concerning the traditional uses of the plants described is from old sources. It is difficult to know if those uses continue today. In many cases, they probably do.

Abies balsamea
Balsam Fir
——
STOP 4

RUSSELL WILLIER

Willier calls this plant *napakâsîta* or Flat-needle Spruce.

Willier uses tea made from the bark for kidney problems. The bark is boiled with other roots to make a combination for treating asthma.

Branches are used to cover the ground at sacred sites such as a sweat lodge.

The Woods Cree call it *napakahsiht* (Flat Branch) or *pikkowahtik* (Gum Wood). The Bush Cree call it a medicine tree, or an infection fighter, *napakâsîta.*

The Cree use the pitch, *napakâsihtipikiw,* for irregular menses and the clear, fragrant resin from the bark to treat cuts, burns, and all manner of skin afflictions. The resin is chewed to relieve heart and chest pains, as well as other respiratory conditions like colds, bronchitis, and asthma. It is combined with sturgeon oil as an ointment to treat tuberculosis. The bark is decocted for kidney and respiratory problems, usually in combination with the roots or bark of other plants. Powdered needles are sprinkled on burns, cuts, and blisters. Even the root is used: small pieces are held in the mouth to relieve sores.

PROPERTIES

Abies and *Picea* species contain a monoterpene, known as isodiprene, which acts as an oxytocin receptor agonist that is anti-inflammatory and induces uterine contractions.

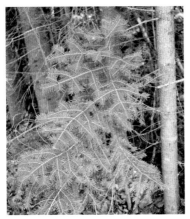 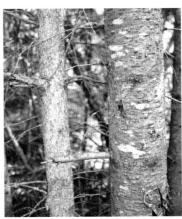

Left: Balsam Fir; Right: A comparison: White Spruce on the left and Balsam Fir on the right (July)

Achillea millefolium
Yarrow
———
STOP 11

RUSSELL WILLIER

Willier calls this plant *wapanowask* or Morning Flower.

Willier uses the flowers of the female plant to treat stings, insect bites, and open sores. He uses the roots in combination with other roots such as Seneca Root for heart problems and chest pains.

Note: What Willier considers to be the male plant is probably *Achillea sibirica*.

ADDITIONAL CREE INFORMATION

Traditionally, the Cree call Yarrow *wapanew-uskwa,* or "bee plant." Cree from different regions have various names for Yarrow: *wapanowask* ("white flower"); *astaweskotawan* ("to put out a campfire" or "burning pain"); *miskigo-nimaski* ("heart medicine"); *mistigonimas-kigah* ("head medicine"); and *osgunim-asgigah* ("bone medicine"). Another Cree name is *amowask.* The Wood Cree call it *ka-wapistikwanikapat.*

The Cree use the entire plant in cold water for burns and for earache. Hot infusions are given to promote menstruation, relieve stomach pain, and control fevers from tuberculosis. Around Lesser Slave Lake, the leaf is infused for late-onset diabetes. The Wood Cree use the dried flowers to disguise the scent of traps used for lynx. Yarrow flower tea or, better yet, the fresh root is rubbed into gums to relieve teething pain. The term "bone medicine" refers to the use in baths or applied as a poultice on affected arthritic areas.

PROPERTIES

The alkamines help to reduce inflammation (Müller-Jakic et al. 1994). This includes reduction of vascular inflammation, noted in work by Dall'Acqua et al. (2011). Matricin, for example, is a propionic acid analog that yields chamazulene carboxylic acid. This compound is a COX-2 inhibitor with activity similar to that of ibuprofen.

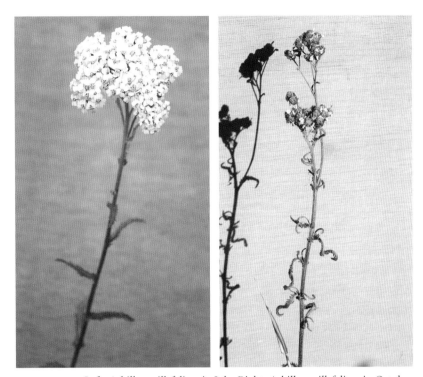

Left: *Achillea millefolium* in July; Right: *Achillea millefolium* in October

Caution: Yarrow should perhaps be avoided during the first trimester of pregnancy due to uterine stimulation from essential oils, but this is questionable. Contraindications are based on a single, low-quality rat study with no significance to humans (Applequist and Moerman 2011). The herb is probably safe for later pregnancy (if there are no heart problems) and during lactation, in small doses. Avoid combining with potassium supplements. Yarrow may interfere with anticoagulant medication (due to coumarin content) and should be avoided by hemophiliacs and perhaps in certain cases of epilepsy. Brinker (2001) believes it may interact with antacids and gastric acid secretion inhibitors, particularly H2-receptor antagonists. In Traditional Chinese Medicine, the herb is not used by those with interior cold, and is used cautiously in those with qi vacuity.

Acorus americanus
Calamus, Sweet Flag, Flagroot

STOP 7

RUSSELL WILLIER

Willier calls this plant *wiyikiyo* or Rat Root.

The root is chewed for strep throat and cough, as well as in combination with other roots such as Seneca Root for heart problems. The root can be stored for at least three years.

ADDITIONAL CREE INFORMATION

The Cree of northern Alberta make great use of this muskrat food—what they call *wachaskomechiwin*. It is also known as Rat Root or Muskrat Root, *wacaskwatapih,* or simply *wihkes* or *wiyikiyo*. The Eastern Ojibwa name is very similar: *wike* or *wee-kees.* The Cree around Hudson Bay call it fire or bitter pepper root, or *pow e men artic.* Gary Raven, a traditional healer from Manitoba, recommends that Calamus, Wild Licorice, and White Water Lily Root be grated and used as a tea to treat diabetes. Small slices can be chewed to treat high cholesterol.

Tis Mal Crow, a Native American root doctor, uses Calamus root as an activator or accelerator that increases the potency of other herbs. He believes it should only be added in one part to thirty-two parts of other herbs, or the mixture may be dangerously strong. Calamus is used specifically with white-flowered medicines for this purpose, violet leaves for green medicines.

PROPERTIES

The asarone-free genotype Calamus shows antispasmodic properties on par with standard antihistamines (Keller et al. 1985). Other Calamus genotypes do not have this property. Work by Gilani et al. (2006) confirms this antispasmodic nature and suggests the activity is calcium channel–like in action. The root is antifungal and antibacterial, but not antiviral, in action. Researchers have identified other compounds in *Acorus calamus* that act on body chemistry other than histamines, to relieve bronchial constriction during asthmatic attacks. Work by

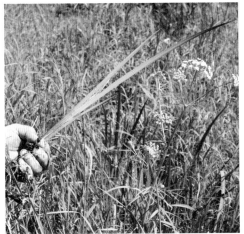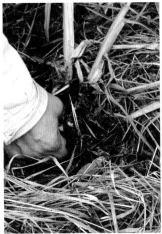

Left: July; Right: October

Acuña et al. (2002) found North American Calamus extracts to possess high levels of antioxidant activity.

Caution: Avoid during pregnancy.

Alnus crispa
Green Alder
———
STOP 2

RUSSELL WILLIER

Willier calls this plant *atôspi* or Hill Willow.

When the tree is flowering and the cones are still green, the cones are used in combinations to treat cancer and to counter hallucinations, curses, and other conditions that result from someone "screwing up." This medicine is a "representative" who talks to the spiritual world on behalf of the healer.

ADDITIONAL CREE INFORMATION

A general Cree name is *atospi* or *miskwatospi*. The Eastern Cree call it *nepatihe*.

The dormant bark is stripped and dried for dying hides that are made into clothing and moccasins. The bark is mixed with animal fats for body paint used in traditional dances. Alder contributes a number of dye colors. The flowers give a green dye, the bark a fiery red, the young shoots cinnamon, and with copper mordant a pure yellow dye is obtained. Eastern Cree use bark decoctions to treat edema. The Cree of northern Saskatchewan boil the green female catkins to treat venereal disease in men. The stems are boiled as an emetic for upset stomach. The root is decocted to relieve menstrual cramps or used as part of a steam/sweat to bring on menstruation.

FOLK USES

The green cones may be tinctured and used for allergies, as well as for bacteria, fungal, and amoebic infections. The freshly dried cones, catkins, leaves, and twigs are tinctured for moving blood and lymphatic fluids (Rogers 2013). Kiva Rose, noted herbalist, writes (2012, 542): "Alder is a staple of my clinical work and one of my most beloved herbal allies. Its consistent and powerful ability to act as a profound alterative and lymphatic while addressing even the most severe microbial infections makes it truly invaluable to almost any practitioner." She notes that Alder does not add to fluids or move or contain them, but transforms their quality. She continues: "I have repeatedly seen cases of staph (including several confirmed cases of MRSA) infection manifesting as repeated outbreaks of boils clear up with the consistent use of Alder tincture."

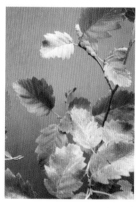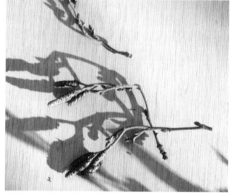

Left: Early Summer; Right: October

Amelanchier alnifolia
Saskatoon

———

STOP 5

RUSSELL WILLIER

Willier calls this plant *saskahtômina* or Saskatoon Berry.

Saskatoon is used in combinations to remove a curse.

ADDITIONAL CREE INFORMATION

Saskatoon appears to originate from the Cree name *missaskwatoomin* or *saskahtômina,* meaning "tree of many branches or wood" or "big berry." Early settlers shortened it to the present name. The name for the city of Saskatoon, Saskatchewan, was derived from the profusion of berry-producing trees in its river valley.

The berries (or pome fruit, to be correct) are prized for use in pies, preserves, ale, and wine. The Native tribes of Alberta store them for winter use, along with Choke Cherries and Blueberries. And of course, it is still a favorite winter browse of moose, deer, and elk. Traditionally, the fruit is sun-dried, either whole or pounded into patties. These Saskatoon loaves weigh up to ten or fifteen pounds. The word "pemmican" may derive from the Cree *pimii* ("fat") and *kan* ("prepared"). It is usually prepared from buffalo meat that was dried and braised over a fire.

The Wood Cree of Saskatchewan use the root as an ingredient in decoctions for teething, chest pain, coughs, and lung infections and to prevent miscarriage. Other tribes use the inner bark to control menstrual flow and as a strengthening tonic both during and after childbirth. The roots and stems are decocted for tuberculosis, while the root is used for coughs and colds, and lung infections of various sorts. Muscle spasms and pinched nerves causing temporary back "paralysis" also benefit from root decoctions. The buds are best boiled for diarrhea, whereas the branch bark is decocted for pleurisy and inflammatory diseases. The Cree combine Snowberry and Saskatoon stem bark in decoction to induce sweating and to treat fevers. In addition, they immerse four to five pieces of barked stem sticks in boiled sturgeon oil for about ten minutes to help keep the oil fresh during storage.

PROPERTIES

Antiviral plant screening at the University of British Columbia by Mc-Cutcheon et al. (1995) showed Saskatoon plant methanol extracts to be very active against enteric bovine coronavirus. This is closely related to respiratory syncytial virus, as both are single-stranded RNA viruses that infect mucous membranes. Work by Kraft et al. (2008) found the nonpolar parts of the fruit inhibit aldose reductase, and moderate expression of IL-1 beta, an anti-inflammatory marker. The polar parts reduce inflammation and improve glucose uptake via an insulin-like effect, suggesting benefit in type-2 diabetes.

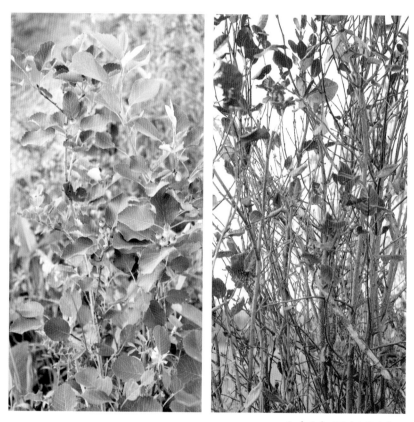

Left: July; Right: October

Angelica genuflexa
Angelica
—
STOP 2

RUSSELL WILLIER

Willier calls this plant *wacaskowîykomawask* or Rat Smell Root.

Roots are used in combinations for cancer, sugar diabetes, high blood pressure, and headaches.

FOLK USES

Sheh Meng Lan et al. (1997) traced the pollen grains of fifty-seven Angelica species from East Asia and North America and found that *A. genuflexa* grows on both continents. White Angelica leaves can be dried and added to barley soups. The seeds can also be collected and dried, making a pleasant celery/cardamom addition to dishes in the wild, or added to potpourri as a fixative. In folk traditions, eating the plant is believed to prevent one from being smelled by bears. The root is a bear medicine, according to the doctrine of signatures, due to its brown, furry, oily, and pungent nature. Other plants of Canada in this category include Lomatium, Wild Licorice, Balsam Root, Devil's Club, Calamus root, and Canby's Lovage.

PROPERTIES

The root is warming, pungent, aromatic, and toning, helping increase circulation to the extremities. The root is considered a specific for Buerger's disease, a condition that inflames and narrows the arteries of the hands and feet. The coumarin, osthol, has been shown to relax guinea pig trachea by inhibiting cyclic AMP and cyclic GMP phosphodiesterases; has a vaso-relaxing effect on thoracic aorta due to calcium blocking properties; and raises levels of cyclic GMP in muscle (Ko et al. 1992). Osthol ameliorates insulin resistance by increment of adiponectin release in high fat and high sugar induced fatty liver rats. Activation of PPAR alpha and gamma pathways are noted (Qi et al. 2011).

Work by Harmala et al. (1991) found archangelicin and other coumarins in the root to be calcium channel antagonists. Imperatorin is an L-type calcium channel blocker that helps to lower blood pressure (Zhang et al. 2011). Vuorela et al. (1997) found archangelicin comparable to Verapamil, a common calcium channel blocker. They work as vasodilators that reduce peripheral vascular resistance. Alpha-angelica lactone, for example, shows anticancer activity in human studies. Psoralens, when taken in isolation, promote tumor growth. And yet whole root extracts show antimutagenic effect in murine bone marrow cell tests (Salikhova and Poroshenko 1995).

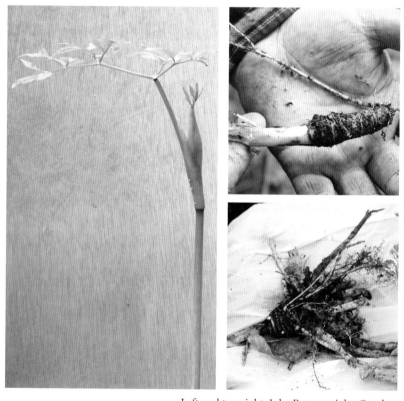

Left and top right: July; Bottom right: October

Caution: Use with care in diabetes or in hot, feverish conditions of any kind. Avoid use with blood thinners such as warfarin due to theoretical interactions with coumarin derivatives in Angelica root. Do not use with cancer drug therapies.

Aralia nudicaulis
Wild Sarsaparilla

STOP 2

RUSSELL WILLIER

Willier calls this plant *waposociyipîyk* or Bear Root.

The root is used in combinations for heart, lungs, liver, and kidneys. The female form of the same species, which is less greasy, is smaller, and has darker green leaves, is called Rabbit Root. It is often combined with Bear Root in combinations. Bear Root is always found under poplar trees.

ADDITIONAL CREE INFORMATION

Compresses of the root, either chewed to a pulp or pounded, are applied to cuts and wounds. It is combined with Labrador Tea and decocted to improve appetite. For children who are teething or have infected gums, the root is crushed and chewed. It is decocted and given whenever pneumonia or other afflictions of the throat and chest occur.

The powdered root is given for venereal disease, probably due to immune-enhancing elements. The fruiting stalk is boiled and tea is given to new mothers to stimulate lactation. Root decoctions are used for childhood pneumonia. Today, various Native healers use it as a preventive for diabetes and cancer. Various Cree healers call it natural Viagra, for its ability to treat impotence.

FOLK USES

Matthew Wood (2009, 70) writes: "The Cree name for *Aralia nudicaulis* translates as 'rabbit root,' according to Rogers. This indicates their conception of the therapeutic direction of the medicine. In the Far North, on the Canadian shield where the Cree live, the rabbit is associated with starvation and emaciation. When the snow is high, only the rabbits can get out on top of the snow, so the deer population dies out and the people have to rely on the rabbit. However, the latter does not provide a complete diet because it lacks good-quality oils. Thus, rabbit medicines are used to antidote the ill-effects of emaciation and atrophy. They are largely nutritive and support the bones and muscles."

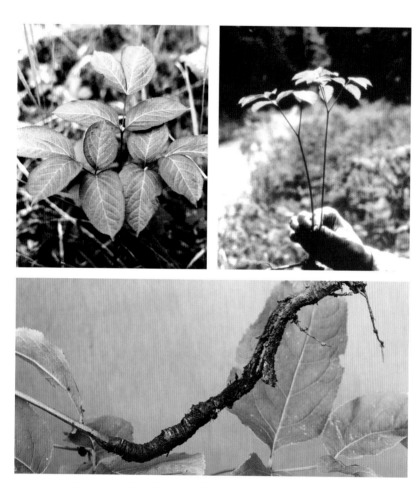

Top photos: Bear Root in early summer (Photographs by research team);
Bottom photo: Rabbit Root (July)

Arbutus menziesii
Arbutus, Madrona, Pacific Madrone

RUSSELL WILLIER

Willier does not have a Cree name for this plant, as it is a recent import from the West Coast of Canada. He uses the English term, Arbutus.

The bark is used in a combination for heart and liver problems, as well as for lowering blood pressure and controlling sugar diabetes.

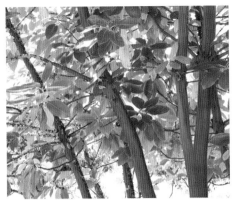 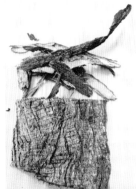

Left: Arbutus in summer; Right: Arbutus bark

ADDITIONAL CREE INFORMATION

Pacific Madrone is a beautiful, monoecious evergreen of western North America. The thin, multilayered bark is red to orange-brown, and later green, red, orange, and brown as it peels with age. The white to pink flowers are sweet and fragrant, and the fruit is a round, orange-red drupe with warty skin that takes a year to mature.

Various coastal tribes used it for stomach ailments, peptic ulcers, burns, cuts, sores and impetigo, and bad colds and for puberty ceremonies. Bark decoctions were generally used as a gargle for strep and sore throats. In the doctrine of signatures or language of plants, the color red represents circulation, and yellow the hepatic system. The peeling layers of bark represent help for skin problems.

Artemisia frigida
Sage, Sagebrush, Prairie Sagewort, Pasture Sage
———
STOP 3

RUSSELL WILLIER

Willier calls this plant *mostoswiyikwaskwa* or Buffalo Grass.

The leaves are used for incense and in many combinations for protection. A very small portion of leaves can be boiled for migraine.

ADDITIONAL CREE INFORMATION

Mostoswiyikiwaska means "good tasting or delicious cow plant." The Cree and others use various Artemisia species for incense and ceremonial purposes. Blackened and weathered leaves were powdered and applied to baby skin rashes, while teas were prepared for stomach complaints.

FOLK USES

The whole plant is infused for bathing. The tincture in cold water reduces stomach hyperacidity. Those troubled by nighttime indigestion or between-meal discomfort will find effective relief. For more chronic cases, Michael Moore (1989) suggests taking the tincture three times daily, in the morning, in the afternoon, and before bed, followed by Alfalfa or Red Clover tea. Vinegar tinctures or well-diluted alcohol tinctures can be applied to the sides of the face and the temples for headaches accompanied by bloodshot eyes. Infusions of the leaves make a good vermifuge. The hot tea is strongly diuretic, and is a moderate laxative for those with atonic constipation. It increases skin secretions, thereby lowering body temperature. Dr. William Cook (1869) recommended warm infusions for their stimulating, diffusive, and diaphoretic properties in malaria, typhoid, rheumatic fever, and scarlatina. It is taken cool for congestive amenorrhea, pelvic engorgements with atony, rheumatism, and diuretic action. The dose is one-half to one drachm in hot lemonade every three hours. Artemisia prefers dry and sandy soil, requiring more southern exposure the further north the plants grow.

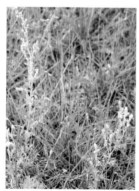 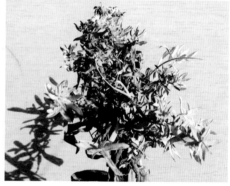

Left: July; Right: October

Aster puniceus
Purple-stemmed Aster, Wild Aster, Aster, Wild Blue Aster

—

STOP 5

RUSSELL WILLIER

Willier calls this plant *misiyistakîyowask, iskomaskiyikêy,* Big Arrow, or Morning Flower.

The root is used in many combinations. A little (no more than three roots) can be boiled and drunk as tea before bed to induce sleep—especially for elders.

ADDITIONAL CREE INFORMATION

The Woods Cree of Saskatchewan call Purple-stemmed Aster either *pawistiko-maskihkih* or *mistahisakwiswask,* meaning "big arrow." The purple lower stem is considered an important indication of the plant's power. In the *Alberta Elders' Cree Dictionary* (LeClaire and Cardinal 1998), Aster is known as a fall or autumn flower, *takwakin wapikwan.*

The Cree use the root for a variety of purposes. Root decoctions are used to induce sweating and to break a fever, as well as after childbirth to help the new mother feel well. It is an ingredient in decoctions for teething and amenorrhea. For toothaches, the root is chewed and applied to the affected area, or mixed with tobacco and smoked for headaches. Roots are used as a diuretic, for cardiac problems, as a medicine for sore kidneys, and for failure to menstruate. Roots are combined with other herbs for insomnia, or in a different combination to ease childbirth pain. The roots are placed on hot rocks in the sweat lodge to make breathing easier and in the treatment of facial paralysis in a condition known as *epimikwipathit* or "twisted face." The aboveground plant is dried and used as a decoction for kidney problems, cold sweats, and chills.

PROPERTIES

The plant has confirmed anti-inflammatory and antispasmodic activity. Various asters show antispasmodic, antitumor, and antiamoebic activity. Many show strong activity against *Mycobacterium tuberculosis.*

The leaves and flowers of various prairie and boreal species are sweet, oily, and aromatic. They tend to be slightly warming and relaxing to the respiratory system, especially with conditions such as irritated coughs and tension asthma. The great eclectic physician, Dr. King (in Ellingwood 1915), had this to say about Purple-stemmed Aster: "Stimulant and diaphoretic. The warm infusion may be used freely in colds, rheumatism, nervous debility, headache, pains in the stomach, dizziness and menstrual irregularities … it has been compared in value with valerian." Valerian is a well-known sedative used for insomnia.

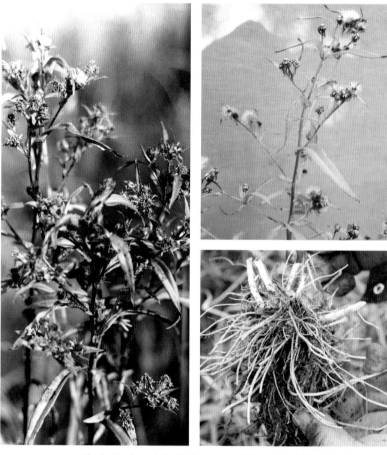

Clockwise from left: Early summer (Photograph by research team);
Fall; Roots in fall

Betula papyrifera
Paper Birch, White Birch

———

STOP 8

RUSSELL WILLIER

Willier calls this plant *waskwiyî* or Birch.

Small sapling stems are used in combinations for blood purification, fever, and conditions of the mind.

ADDITIONAL CREE INFORMATION

The white rotten wood is boiled by the Cree with Labrador Tea. This extract was dried and powdered and used as a dusting powder on chapped skin. The dry, powdered rotten wood was used as baby powder. For gonorrhea, the buds are used, whereas for lung trouble, bark infusions are combined with Hemlock or Spruce. The Cree of northern Manitoba collect Birch bark from the east side of the tree, and boil it with another plant for women who cannot conceive. The Cree of Alberta used the tree bark traditionally for baskets, canoes, bowls, and moose callers. The fall wood is used for making snowshoes good for dry snow. When the snow is wet, these snowshoes absorb too much moisture and become too heavy. Small-diameter trees with bark left on are ideal for woodworking files and other handles, as they do not split. Birch wood is also used to make toboggans, drum frames, canoe paddles, and hide stretching racks. Moose calls from rolled Birch have been found in Mesolithic North American caves. Birch bark can be tightly wrapped and tied with Dogbane twine as a wilderness torch. It burns intensely and bright but tends to drop ash.

FOLK USES

The Birch juice, derived from fresh Birch leaves, is an efficient blood cleanser, with a stimulating effect on the kidneys. It offers relief in the treatment of rheumatic and other swollen, inflamed conditions. The wet, internal side of fresh Birch bark gives quick external relief to rheumatic pain. When decocted, the fresh Birch bark turns a beautiful rose color.

The water is strained and used as a fomentation for skin rash, dermatitis, and cradle cap, and on the elderly with paper-thin skin. Internally, when cooled, the inner-bark decoction will help resolve boils. Taken cold, before bedtime, it will help relieve night sweats (Rogers 2014).

PROPERTIES

Betulin has been found to activate GABA(A) receptor sites, suggesting use in anxiety or depressive mental states (Muceniece et al. 2008). Recent work suggests the use of betulinic acid against a variety of human cancer cell lines (Fulda 2008). Birch bark standardized extracts at 160 milligrams daily were given to forty-two patients with chronic hepatitis C for twelve weeks. Fatigue and abdominal pain reduced sixfold, and aspartate aminotransferase by 54 percent (Shikov et al. 2011). Birch bark has been found, *in vivo*, to possess antitumor activity against B16, sarcoma 180, and Lewis lung cancer cell lines (Han et al. 2000).

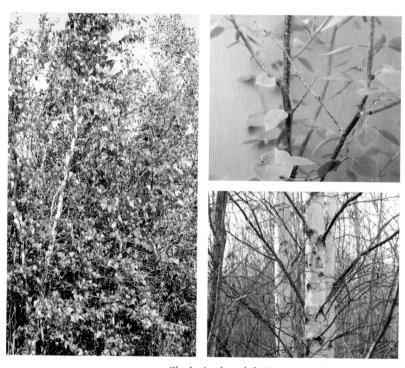

Clockwise from left: Summer; Early summer; Fall

Betula pumila or *B. nana*
Bog Birch, Dwarf Birch, Swamp Birch

STOP 8

RUSSELL WILLIER

Willier calls this plant *apistiwaskwayi* or Small Birch.

Willier uses Bog and Swamp Birch in the same ways as Paper Birch, especially when Paper Birch cannot be found.

ADDITIONAL CREE INFORMATION

Bog Birch produces cones in the fall, which are combined with Labrador Tea by the Cree of Alberta for pneumonia. Other Cree healers say to boil the stems and leaves of Bog Birch as weight-loss tea. The twig tips are decocted to stop both internal and external bleeding. The name, Bog Birch, is unfortunate, as the shrub is rarely found in bogs, but is more often found in fen-like situations, Black Spruce swamps, and alpine slopes. The Cree of northern Manitoba collect Birch bark from the east side of the tree, and boil it with another plant for women who cannot conceive. The twig tips can be decocted to stop both internal and external bleeding.

FOLK USES

Swamp Birch (*B. pumila*) cones can be set on low coals and inhaled for

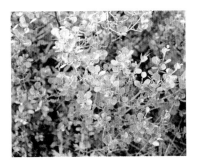

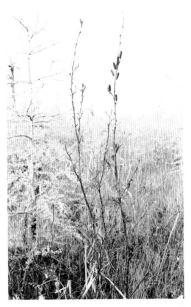

Top: Early summer; Bottom: Fall

severe and chronic sinus inflammations. It is sometimes difficult to distinguish between Bog and Swamp Birch. Generally, Swamp Birch is taller, up to 2–3 meters, whereas Bog Birch may reach 150 centimeters. They both contain resin glands, but Swamp Birch leaves have a very distinct reddish tinge on the underside.

Castilleja raupii
Indian Paintbrush or Red Paintbrush

—

STOP 1

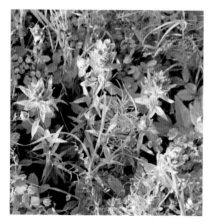 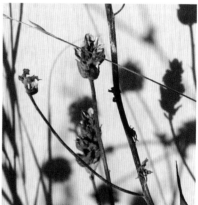

RUSSELL WILLIER

Willier calls this plant *okimawask* or King Root.

It is used in combinations to remove a curse and for protection.

FOLK USES

The Paintbrushes are all semi-parasitic, which stands them in good stead in times of stress and drought. The showy leaf bracts look like a Paintbrush, hence the common name. This particular red-pink species has an affinity for south-facing slopes with good drainage. The flowers can be eaten, and in particular, the long corolla tubes are rich in nectar. The flowers and tea are used in love medicines.

Cicuta maculata
Spotted Water Hemlock, Cowbane
———
STOP 10

RUSSELL WILLIER

Willier calls this plant *manitoskâtâsk* or God's Carrot.

Willier uses a very small portion of the root in a combination for cancer. This is a very dangerous medicine, used by some for curses.

ADDITIONAL CREE INFORMATION

The Woods Cree of Saskatchewan know Water Hemlock as *maciskatask,* meaning "bad carrot." The root was dried, powdered, and made into a liniment that was applied externally. The Cree of Alberta call it *manitoskâtâsk,* or "poison carrot." Small amounts of the root are used in cancer combinations. John Richardson ([1832] 1991) wrote of Water Hemlock that the poisonous kinds are called *manitoskatash,* and by the voyageurs "Carotte de Moreau," or Carrot of Death, after a man died from eating them.

PROPERTIES

Cicutoxin is a potent, noncompetitive GABA-receptor antagonist. Religious sects of the fifteenth and sixteenth centuries used roasted poison hemlock root externally to relieve the pain of gout, not only on the foot, but in hands and wrists. In the 1700s, it was used for curing cancerous ulcers. The juice of poison hemlock is still valued by druggists. Coniine and other alkaloids are extracted from the leaves and young shoots, just as the fruits form. Coniine is a paralysis-inducing nAChR agonist and a toxic teratogenic compound. Cicutoxin is a potent K+ current blocker that inhibits K+ channel dependent proliferation of naive and memory T lymphocytes (Rogers 2014). In homeopathic form (small doses), the root is used for breast cancer.

Caution: Do not ingest the fresh or dried plant. If ingested, use morphine and thiobarbiturates to control convulsions. When seizures have occurred, do not attempt gastric lavage without an anesthesiologist present. Prolonged mental problems and irregular ECGs have been reported. It is the antidote for strychnine poisoning, as its activity is directly antagonistic.

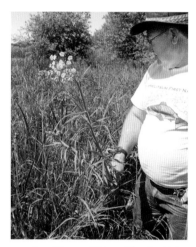

Cicuta maculata (Spotted Water Hemlock) in summer

Compare this dangerous plant with *Heracleum lanatum* in the next photograph. Even though the flowers are similar, Spotted Water Hemlock has narrow leaves whereas the leaves of Cow Parsnip are broad.

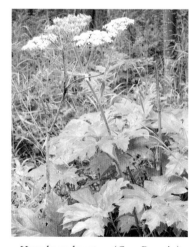

Heracleum lanatum (Cow Parsnip)

Cornus stolonifera
Red Osier Dogwood
——
STOP 1

RUSSELL WILLIER

Willier calls this plant *mikwapimakwa* or Red Willow.

Willier boils the top four inches of fresh growth for energy and as a blood tonic. It can be picked any time of the year. Berries are used to break a love charm. The bark is used as a tobacco substitute.

ADDITIONAL CREE INFORMATION

The *Alberta Elders' Cree Dictionary* (LeClaire and Cardinal 1998) name for this plant is *mihkwapemakwa ka pihtwat-amihk*. Other variations are *mihkwâpimakomina*, "dog berry"; *mikwapanuk, mehkwa pemakwa, mikobimaka, mikwapimakwa*, "red willow"; *mikwapiskaw,* "red wood"; and *mehkwapemak,* "red stem."

The Cree use *mihkwapimakwahtik* (meaning "dog wood") stem bark tea for chest troubles, coughs, and fevers. Stem tea, consumed cool, is taken for dysuria, the inability to urinate. The white berries are used for tuberculosis and externally as a wash for snow blindness, whereas the pith of branches is used for cataracts. Dogwood inner bark is a sedative and is useful for insomnia. The hardly tasty white berries are combined with ripe Saskatoon berries, and called "sweet and sours." The Cree use the inner bark as a tobacco, part of *kinnickinnick,* or "smoking mixture." The bitter outer red bark is removed, and the inner bark was then curled back six or eight inches in clusters, the sharp end stuck in the ground near a fire and roasted until dry. The fine scrapings of the inner bark are used to cure coughs and fevers or induce vomiting as necessary. Finely ground and powdered bark is used as a styptic for bleeding and for wounds that refuse to heal.

FOLK USES

The leaves can be dried and used as a tobacco substitute. The stems make excellent smoking pipe stems by pushing the soft pith from the center of the hard stems. Goldenrod galls contain a white larva that is

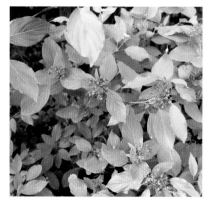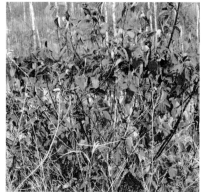

Left: Early summer; Right: Fall

placed into one end of the cut stem and sealed in. The insect has no choice but to transit the entire length to exit, thus creating a perfect pipe stem for those with time to wait. Dream catchers are often made from Dogwood, due to its connection with dreams and charms. The ripe, white berry juice is a wonderful hair conditioner (Rogers 2014).

Corylus cornuta
Hazelnut

—

STOP 9

RUSSELL WILLIER

Willier calls this plant *pakanâhtihk* or Peanut Willow.
  It is used in combinations to remove curses.

ADDITIONAL CREE INFORMATION

The Cree call the bush *pakanâhtihk,* and the nut *pakan.* They use the twig tea for treating heart disease. Some Native people bury the harvested nuts until the husks rot, by filling the hole with wet mud for up to ten days. After removing the husks, the nuts are shelled and eaten, or stored for later use. The Eastern Cree make a tea of the branch tips to cure heart troubles. Young, straight shoots were prepared by Natives of the Canadian prairies for arrows, snowshoes, and drumming sticks. They twist the peeled shoots to break the fiber and use them as plied rope for lashing and tying.

FOLK USES

Gloves are a must in harvesting, due to the rough husk, but if the skin is irritated, simply rub fresh leaves on the inflamed area. This green husk is quite salty when chewed, indicating another possible source of land-locked sodium salts from plant ash. The smaller, immature nuts still in the milky stage are soft and sweet. They can be picked this way before the squirrels start to gather them. Spoons are carved from the wood, as it does not have a strong flavor. A blue dye, for coloring baskets, is made from the buds or roots when scraped and exposed to air. This can be rubbed on, or a decoction made by soaking either part in water. The leaves are diuretic and useful for varicose veins and circulatory problems, usually as a hot infusion, or as an extract. The hot leaves are poulticed as a vein tonic, the astringency helping to shrink the tissues.

PROPERTIES

Hazelnut contains paclitaxel in the twigs, leaves, kernels, and shells of the nut. Paclitaxel, the active ingredient in the antican-cer drug Taxol, is a taxane found in Yew trees of the *Taxus* species. Taxol, as a drug, has been approved for the treatment of ovarian and breast cancers, as well as non-small-cell lung cancer. It may be of possible benefit in psoriasis, polycystic kidney

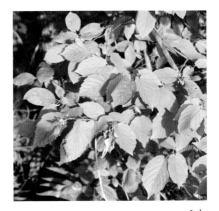

July

disease, and Alzheimer's disease. Recent research at St. Michael's Hospital in Toronto indicates paclitaxel may have application in the treatment of multiple sclerosis. Micellar paclitaxel, which is a soluble form, appears to curb an enzyme that damages the myelin sheath. When damaged, it is harder for nerves to transmit signals to the rest of the body. No tests have been conducted on Hazelnut twig extracts, but considering the relative safety, this would be worth a trial.

Dryopteris carthusiana
Narrow Spinulose Shield Fern

STOP 6

RUSSELL WILLIER

Willier calls this plant *wiyinohwask* or Fat Root.

The middle, green part of the root is boiled and eaten, or the liquid drunk, to treat worms and to help people gain weight by giving them a strong appetite. Willier also uses Shield Fern in combinations for cancer.

ADDITIONAL CREE INFORMATION

The Cree of northern Alberta call all ferns by the generic name *masanahtik*. The Cree know *Dryopteris carthusiana* as raven's beak or *ku(h)kuguwpuk*.

FOLK USES

The pineapple-like rhizomes are dug up in fall, when they are surrounded with the scaly fingers of next year's growth. They can be picked in spring before new ferns emerge, but this makes them harder to find. If dark and flat inside, the rhizome is not used for food, but if light colored and fleshy, it is steamed in pits or boiled over a fire, tasting similar to a sweet potato or yam. A favorite meal is made by peeling the rootstocks after cooking, and then smearing them with grease or fermented fish eggs. The roots, for food, are best in spring or fall. Various *Dryopteris* roots are used for toothache, worms, and other intestinal complaints. Ointment from the root heals ulcerous and cancerous tumors. This includes Spiny Wood Fern, which was used medicinally as well as for food. Shield Fern is used to make infusions for dandruff. The roots are decocted and used as foot baths in treating varicose veins. Mature fronds are stuffed in linen bags for rheumatism. The root is thrown into the fire at the summer solstice as a power charm. Some Natives eat the uncurled fronds before a hunt, to help mask their scent. The curled shoots of Shield Fern are taken as part of a compound decoction as an appetite stimulant. The frond stipe bases have been traditionally decocted with other herbs for kidney pain, in other mixtures for skin washes, as cancer therapy, or smoked with other plants to treat "insanity."

Caution: The fern root should not be administered in the presence of anemia; cardiac, liver, or kidney disease; or diabetes. It is not advisable for children, during pregnancy, or for the elderly. Overdose can lead to central nervous system disorders like spasm, paralysis, visual disorders, and even blindness. Benzodiazepines and oxygen may be needed in case of seizure or respiratory failure.

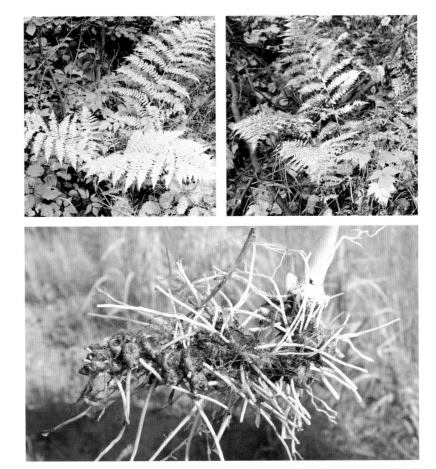

Clockwise from top left: Early summer; Fall; Fall

Elaeagnus commutata
Wolf Willow
———
STOP 13

RUSSELL WILLIER

Willier calls this plant *soniyawniyipsi* or Silver Willow.
It is used in combinations to remove a curse.

ADDITIONAL CREE INFORMATION

The plant is known in Cree as either *wapi-wuskwa-mepise* or *soniyawniyipsi*.
The Cree use the silver fruit in soups or as decorative beads. Northern Cree use the tough inner bark for weaving baskets, and as rope for nets, fishing line, and even clothing.

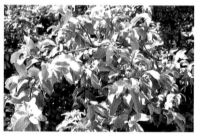

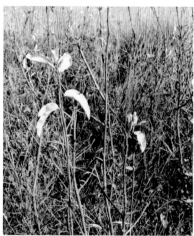

Top: Early summer; Bottom: Fall

FOLK USES

To make the seeds usable, they are first boiled and when soft, the holes are drilled. They are then threaded, dried, oiled, and polished. The root bark is stronger than trunk bark, but both remain flexible after drying. The inner bark is dried for future use and, when needed, soaked in water and spun into a strong, two-ply twine, or larger if desired. A favorite campfire practical joke is to secretly add a twig of Wolf Willow to the blaze and watch everyone's accusatory reactions to the excrement-smelling smoke.

Epilobium angustifolium (*Chamerion angustifolium*)
Fireweed

—

STOP 2

RUSSELL WILLIER

Willier calls this plant *eskohtiyowaskwa, skohtiyôciyipihk,* or Fireweed. The roots are used to purify the blood.

ADDITIONAL CREE INFORMATION

The Cree call it *ihkapaskwa,* and note that it flowers when the moose are fattening and mating. Other names include *askapask, athkapask,* and *akapuskwah.*

The root is macerated and applied to boils or skin infections. The leaves are plastered on bruises. The raw roots are a popular Native food source. Even the summer stem was split open with the thumbnail or between the teeth, to extract the inner edible "pith." It tastes a bit like cucumber but is very sweet and can give a sugar buzz when needed. The Woods Cree of Saskatchewan make a tea of the whole plant for intestinal parasites. The root can be crushed and applied to boils or abscesses, or used to draw out infection from open wounds. The root is used by the Cree of Wabasca as part of a decoction to reveal whether or not a woman is pregnant. If the decoction, when drunk, causes a violent nosebleed, she's pregnant. Otherwise, menstruation will begin.

FOLK USES

The fluff from ripened pods is used as tinder to start fires, and when carbonized is extremely susceptible to the smallest spark or heat friction. "Wick up" refers to the use of rolled fluff as a wilderness candlewick inserted in tallow or other fat. Its insulating factor has been utilized as fiber combined with mountain goat hair to make blankets. Other Natives used duck feather/Cattail/Fireweed combinations. Down feathers and Fireweed fluff make excellent comforters. It also makes an excellent wilderness bandage combined with Balsam Fir pitch. In an experiment by Salisbury (1961), Fireweed fluff was dropped ten feet in a draft-free room. It took the better part of a minute to sail to the floor, explaining its wide dispersion in nature.

PROPERTIES

Work by Vitali et al. (2006) found topical applications analgesic and anti-inflammatory, and internal use antidiarrheal and antimotile on gastrointestinal tissue. The aerial parts have a long tradition of use in reducing benign prostatic hyperplasia. Kiss et al. (2004) found Fire-weed extracts inhibitory against angiotensin-converting enzyme, aminopeptidase N, and neutral endopeptidase (NEP), all of which play a role in prostate disease. The rhizomes contain fewer tannins, and no mucilage, but contain the flavonoids useful for the anti-inflammatory process in treating conditions such as prostatitis and enlarged prostate (Rogers 2014).

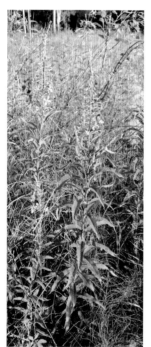
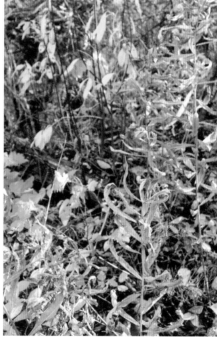

Left: Early summer; Right: Fall

Fragaria virginiana
Wild Strawberry

STOP 8

RUSSELL WILLIER

Willier calls this plant *ohtihmina* or Heart Berry.

The roots are boiled with Yarrow to make a tea for insanity and diarrhea. The root is also used for the heart.

ADDITIONAL CREE INFORMATION

The Cree call Wild Strawberry *otiyihimina,* or heart berry.

To help cure "insanity," they boil the roots and those of Yarrow together, and drink it cool. For heart conditions, the leaves or roots are decocted for forty-five minutes, and the tea is allowed to cool. For diarrhea, the roots, leaves, and runners are all boiled, sometimes combined with Yarrow. For healing open sores, an ash made by burning the roots can be mixed into a paste.

FOLK USES

Leaf and stem tea can be gargled for sore throats, and used to relieve the itch of vaginal or yeast infections, and to shrink hemorrhoids with external bathing. The leaf is often used in combinations for liver disease, jaundice, respiratory congestion, gout, rheumatoid arthritis, and kidney complaints involving stones or gravel. The leaf tea acidifies urine and may help urinary tract infections associated with alkalinity. The leaf relieves irritable bowel and colitis, when taken as a cooled infusion. The root is stronger and needs decoction. Both stomach and intestinal hyperacidity are relieved. Infused roots are taken to dry up breast milk in women trying to wean babies. It diminishes the size of breasts and dries up the milk. A root and leaf infusion helps diarrhea and summer complaint in children. A fluid extract commercial product on the market was originally produced from the root and is still widely sold. The root is very astringent, and holding it in the mouth will help stop nosebleeds (Rogers 2014). The liver is assisted by the increased protein breakdown, which in turn helps alleviate allergies.

PROPERTIES

McCutcheon et al. (1992) found Wild Strawberry leaves contain antibiotic activity against seven of eleven bacterial strains, including MRSA (methicillin-resistant *Staphylococcus aureus*) and *Pseudomonas aeruginosa.* Activity against *E. coli* was equal to that of gentamicin. The leaf showed moderate antifungal activity on seven of nine species (McCutcheon et al. 1994).

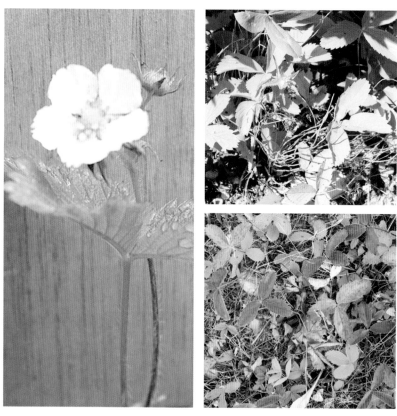

Clockwise from left: Early summer;
Early summer, Fall (photo by Robert Rogers)

Gaultheria hispidula
Creeping Wintergreen

STOP 8

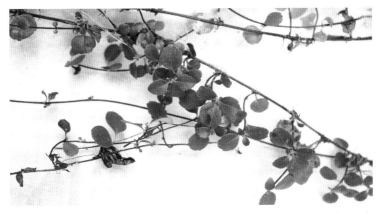

Summer

RUSSELL WILLIER

Willier calls this plant *apstepakosa* or Tiny Leaves.

Leaves are used in combinations to make tea for high fever, for high blood pressure, and as a tobacco substitute.

ADDITIONAL CREE INFORMATION

The Cree call it *apschiypukos* or *apstepakosa,* meaning "tiny leaves."

The Cree around Wabasca, near Lesser Slave Lake, use leaf decoctions to treat hypertension. They combine the leaves with other herbs, such as Yarrow, to treat fevers, or simply add them to tea for a pleasant flavor. The cooled decoction soothes teething pains in young babies. Eastern Cree use the leaf tea for headaches and colds, or as part of a chest plaster for asthma. During the nineteenth century, the stem tea was recommended for morning sickness.

PROPERTIES

Gaultherin is a conjugated salicylate, with a disaccharide. Methyl salicylate is released from gaultherin after hydrolysis of the disaccharide by gaultherase in plants, or other hydrolases in humans. Salicylic acid is then formed by the removal of the methyl ester by ubiquitous esterases. This suggests Wintergreen may provide a time-release form of pharmacologically active salicylate and a safer, natural alternative to aspirin. More than fifteen million people in the United States alone take aspirin on a regular basis for cardiac health and cancer prevention (Ribnicky et al. 2003).

Caution: Do not take with blood thinners. Individuals with salicylate sensitivity should use with caution. Do not use during pregnancy or lactation (Rogers 2014).

Geum aleppicum or *G. macrophyllum*
Yellow Avens, Large-leaved Yellow Avens

STOP 11

RUSSELL WILLIER

Willier calls this plant *sakohtowask* or Jealousy Root (or Love Root).

It is used for sexual prowess and in combinations for a variety of ailments. The plant is ground up and added to other herbs for medicine or used as a smudge under a blanket.

Note: Smaller plants (perhaps female, in Willier's opinion) may be what he calls Court Medicine (*weasuwilmuskegi*), used to help the healer foresee what will happen in court to someone who has been framed.

ADDITIONAL CREE INFORMATION

Yellow and Large-leaved Yellow Avens are known as *kakwithitamowask* or "jealousy plant." This is due to the achenes hooking onto the clothing of passersby—just like when a person is walking by and someone is jealous of them. It is also called *saw gee too wusk*.

The Woods Cree of Saskatchewan decoct the root alone or in combination to treat sickness associated with teething and to induce sweating. Decoctions are used for sore teeth or for sore throats.

FOLK USES

The various native Avens roots are one of the better Cree remedies for dysentery and chronic diarrhea. It is a good remedy for bloody or odorous vaginal discharge, using the cooled decocted tea as a douche. For hemorrhoids, a retention enema works wonders. In addition, it will help to stop uterine hemorrhages, excessive menstruation. and middle-of-the-month bleeding like Cranesbill, a geranium native to North America. Avens is a good tea for irritation and inflammation of the stomach lining, and even ulcerative colitis, using either the dried leaf or stronger root tea. Large-leaved Avens fresh root tincture helps reduce fevers, in the manner of quinine. Use one-half to one teaspoon in warm water every hour until improved. This same tincture can help improve and regulate liver and gallbladder function. It combines well with Angelica root and Silverweed root as a stomach tonic. Dig the root as early in the spring as possible (Rogers 2000).

PROPERTIES

Studies conducted by McCutcheon et al. (1992, 1994) at the University of British Columbia found that *G. macrophyllum* root is a great fungal inhibitor and showed activity against nine of eleven bacteria tested, especially *E. coli.*

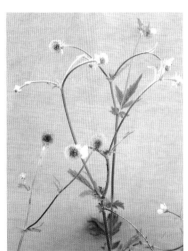 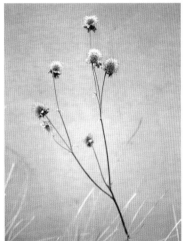

Left: Early summer; Right: Fall

Geum rivale
Purple Avens, Water Avens

———

STOP 1

RUSSELL WILLIER

Willier calls this plant *kiniyipikominanatihk* or Snake Root.

The root is boiled and used to increase sexual prowess and to help with difficult childbirth.

ADDITIONAL CREE INFORMATION

The Cree call this plant *kinipagwask* or *kinipagwuskhas,* meaning "snake root."

It was traditionally decocted for unwanted pregnancy.

FOLK USES

Chocolate root, as it is sometimes known, is used for fevers and diarrhea as well. A cocoa substitute is made from the root, hence the name, and it is used as a tonic.

PROPERTIES

G. rivale leaves and roots show activity against gram-negative and gram-positive bacteria, as well as fungi (Panizzi et al. 2000), probably due to triterpene and/or flavonoid content. Water Avens was written about extensively by Dr. Cook (1869): "Its action on the duodenum and mesenteries fits it for a class of cases to which few articles are applicable; and I am decidedly of the opinion that it will be found useful in *tabes mesenterica,* and in those forms of scrofulous looseness of the bowels which are dependent upon defective assimilation, and which often pass roughly as chronic diarrhea. This distinction between tonics to the digestive and to the assimilative apparatus, is one that has not heretofore been made; but it is one of importance, and those which act on the assimilative organs are so few as to deserve especial notice."

Lucinda Haynes Lombard, writing for *The American Botanist* in November 1918, noted a peculiar superstition: friends provided with *G.*

rivale leaves are able to converse with one another though many miles apart and speaking in whispers, suggestive of telepathy.

Homeopathic Water Avens (*G. rivale*) is for severe jerking pains from deep in the abdomen to the end of the urethra. It is for infections of the bladder with pains in the penis. They are like electric shocks, always occurring twice in succession. The symptoms are made worse by eating, with imperfect digestion and assimilation. Excessive and depraved secretions, and relaxed mucous membranes, are other symptoms.

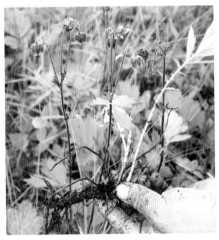

Early summer

Grindelia squarrosa
Gumweed

STOP 3

RUSSELL WILLIER

Willier calls this plant *kapikiyowapakwani* or Gum Flower.

The stems and blossoms are burned and the smoke breathed in for migraine headache. It is also used to treat venereal disease.

ADDITIONAL CREE INFORMATION

The Cree call it *kah-pus-kun-askik, kapasakwask maskihkih,* or *kapiki-yowapakwani.*

They use the entire plant with Pineapple Weed (*Matricaria discoidea*) for kidney pain, and buds and flowers only for gonorrhea. The plant was used by women in an unspecified manner to prevent pregnancy.

FOLK USES

Gumweed is a circulatory stimulant and respiratory relaxant, or anti-spasmodic. Gumweed relaxes the smooth and swollen bronchi as well as heart muscle. This makes it invaluable in asthmatic and bronchial conditions where there is a rapid heartbeat and nervous response. Gumweed therefore combines well with Sundew for whooping cough, or whenever increased expectoration is called for. One of the key symptoms is dry, spasmodic coughing, but also excessive thick and sticky phlegm that is difficult to remove. It softens and moisturizes the bronchi, increasing mucolytic activity. A strong, hot infusion of half cider and half water helps loosen a cough and relax the lungs. It helps to desensitize nerve endings in the bronchial tree and slow heart rate (Rogers 2014).

Ellingwood (1915) writes: "Dr. Webster is the authority for the statement that *Grindelia squarrosa* is specific in its antimalarial properties. He is very positive concerning its influence upon headaches and especially those of malarial origin. Headache present where there are masked intermittent symptoms, headache accompanied with dizziness and some nausea, where the subject walks with the sensation that he is going to stagger. It seems as though his equilibrium were uncertain, or where there is mild staggering and irregular gait, where the head feels light and dizzy all the time. In this form, *Grindelia squarrosa* is a positive and specific remedy, decided and satisfactory in its action."

Another form of headache this agent will cure is one that seems to follow and depend upon slow autointoxication. It is persistent, day after day, and there is dullness, drowsiness, and dizziness. There is apt to be torpor of the liver and spleen in these cases. There is lassitude, and the patient tires easily. A dull headache is present when he awakes in the morning and with some exacerbations continues all day. This form is quickly cured with this remedy. A tincture made by covering the fresh plant with 98 percent alcohol is required to relieve this headache. Give from ten to fifteen drops of this tincture every two or three hours.

Caution: Grindelia has the capacity to take up and store selenium from the soil. Many parts of the northern plains are selenium deficient, but in large doses selenium is toxic, even the organic type. Because the active principles are excreted through the kidneys, it will initially raise blood pressure and heart rate, and then lower them. Use recommended doses. Large amounts of tincture can cause mild symptoms of exhaustion, according to Michael Moore (1989). Do not use during pregnancy, or for those with weak hearts. Excessive dosage irritates the kidneys (Rogers 2003).

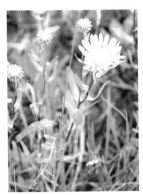 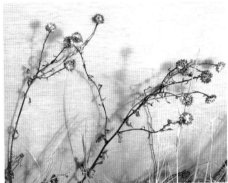

Left: Early summer; Right: Fall

Haploporus odorus
Diamond Willow Fungus

STOP 2

RUSSELL WILLIER

Willier calls this plant *wikiyimakasikan* or Diamond Willow Fungus. This white fungus is found on willow trees more than fifty years old.

It can grow on more than one species of willow, though primarily on Diamond Willow. It is used in purification ceremonies.

ADDITIONAL CREE INFORMATION

The Cree call it *wiy(h)kimasiygan* or *wasaskwetiw*.

Diamond Willow Fungus has a great deal of special significance to the Native people of the northern plains and boreal forest. It grows specifically on Diamond Willow, and the fungus size is directly related to the diameter of its host tree. It is smudged, as part of special ceremonies, and with its special coumarin/anise-like odor, is very pleasing to the mind and body. It is a special gift given to healers conducting sweat lodges, as the fungus is believed to guard and protect against unseen forces. The smoke is used in blessings and as part of cleansing and empowerment events. It was traditionally used to decorate sacred robes, as a symbol of spiritual power, and was found in medicine bundles. It is considered to have protective powers, and when taken in infusion will stop diarrhea and dysentery, or it can be combined in decoction with Indian Breadroot (*Psoralea esculenta*) to treat coughs.

FOLK USES

The smoke is inhaled for treating headaches, or the fresh conk squeezed for juice for earaches. It is a styptic for wounds, making it very valuable in both accidents and battle. It is often used as a mosquito smudge when camping in summer. It definitely adds a brightened and vivid element to the dream state. Large specimens make good gifts to elders and spiritual leaders. The smoke is inhaled through the nostrils twice and repeated every five to ten minutes in cases of migraine headache. The benefit in many cases is long lasting. The white fungus worn around necks, about the size of tennis balls, has been mistakenly assumed in the past to be puffballs. In fact, this was carved Diamond Willow Fungus. It is also found attached to robes and blankets (Rogers 2011).

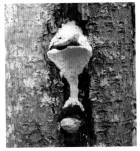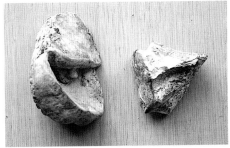

Left: Growing on Diamond Willow; Right: After drying

Heracleum lanatum
Cow Parsnip

STOP 2

RUSSELL WILLIER

Willier calls this plant *pakwânâhtik* or Empty Stalk. The root is used in combinations for cancer. Powdered roots make a poultice for boils or glandular swelling. The stem is used as a siphon to drink water when one can't bend over. Seeds are used on guns to make them shoot straight. The stem can be eaten but it must be peeled first or it will cause blisters.

ADDITIONAL CREE INFORMATION

The Cree call this plant *pukwan-ahtik* or "tent-like leaf wood" or "tent wood." It is also called *piygwanatik* or *pagwanatik*, meaning "hollow inside." Another Cree name is *manitoskatask*. The Cree of Saskatchewan call it *askiwiskatask* or "earth carrot."

The Cree apply the mashed roots to boils or glandular swellings. Small pieces of the root are applied to sore teeth, and the poison collected was spit out with the juice. The root is combined with Calamus and Water Lily Root for external relief from painful limbs or severe headaches.

FOLK USES

The stems, when cooked and limp, taste like celery with a rhubarb texture. They are more than 18 percent protein and full of nourishment.

The stems contain furanocoumarins that can cause photosensitivity in some individuals. Use gloves to gather. The stems are best before flowering, later becoming more bitter. The stem is split open and then bent back upon itself to separate the stringy outer peel from the edible and fleshy inner portion. Peeling the stems helps prevent this sensitivity. Some Native people believe the plants growing in shade are edible, whereas those in full sun should be avoided, probably due to this phototoxicity. The peeled stalks contain only half the furanocoumarins. The hollow tubes were filled with animal blood, dried, and stored for winter. The roots are mashed, when fresh, or roasted over hot coals, and taste like turnip or sweet potatoes. The first-year roots are most tasty and the least trouble. Mors Kochanski compares the small internal roots to ginseng in flavor (personal communication). The raw root may be poulticed and applied to swollen glands, or combined with water as a gargle for sore throats. The dried green seeds possess antiviral and antispasmodic properties useful for trigeminal neuralgia, Bell's palsy, and various types of nerve-related paralysis of head and neck (Rogers 2014).

Caution: The fresh stems and leaves contain hairs and sap that will severely burn sensitive people. It will also cause light sensitivity to affected areas.

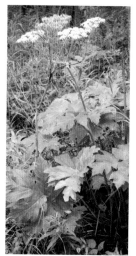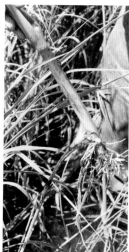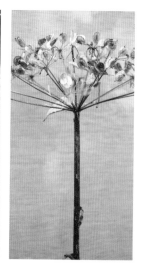

Left and center: Early summer; Right: Fall

Also avoid use during pregnancy or lactation due to sterol and saponin content. Vinegar and water seem to antidote the blotches and blisters.

Hierochloe odorata (*Anthoxanthum nitens*)
Sweet Grass

STOP 11

RUSSELL WILLIER

Willier calls this plant *wêkaskwa* or Sweet Grass.

Plants are braided and used for purification. The tips are put in water when praying or in combinations to speak on behalf of the healer.

ADDITIONAL CREE INFORMATION

The Northern Cree know it as *wiyikaskwa,* sweet scented grass, while other Cree call it *wehkuskwa,* or shorten the name to *wekus.* It is known to the Woods Cree of Saskatchewan and the Northern Cree of Alberta as *wakinakan* or *waginatik,* meaning "bends easily." The Cree in Saskatchewan boil four sweet grass braids and give the decoction to a young girl suffering difficult labor to speed up and assist childbirth.

FOLK USES

Sweet Grass is burned for its spiritually purifying and protective properties. Woven strands are symbols of life's growth and renewing powers. Kahlee Keane (2003) writes "in plaiting a braid, the three sections signify mind, body and spirit." Sacred pipes or hunting weapons are all passed through the smoke for strength. In some Native legends, the fairies were so mesmerized by their own reflections in a pool that they pined away, leaving only the memory of their sweet scent lingering upon the grass. The leaves are mixed with tobacco and smoked to summon the benevolent power possessed by sweet grass. It is even braided into the hair, or soaked in water to make a hair wash. The stems are soaked in water to wash chapped and wind-burned skin or to treat sore eyes. Sweet Grass is mixed with the gelatin of boiled hooves as a hair tonic.

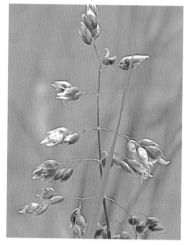 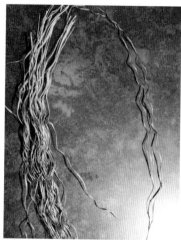

Left: July (Photo by Robert Rogers); Right: Before braiding

PROPERTIES

Sweet Grass aerial parts contain at least two compounds with free-radical scavenging activity (Pukalskas et al. 2002).

Larix laricina
Tamarack

STOP 1

RUSSELL WILLIER

Willier calls this plant *wakanakahn* or Bendable Stem.

The bark is used in combinations for cleansing the throat and blood. The bark is also used on open sores to suck out poison and infections. It can be used to treat tuberculosis.

ADDITIONAL CREE INFORMATION

The Cree make tea from the inner bark to wash skin sores, burns, frost-bite and wounds, as well as hemorrhoids, ear and eye inflammations, jaundice, and colic. Internally the tea is used to relieve melancholy. The Woods Cree of Saskatchewan use the inner bark as a poultice to heal

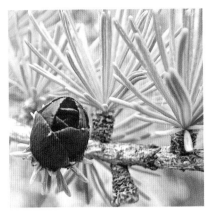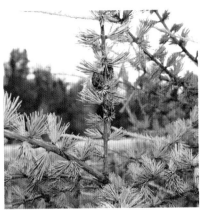

Left: Spring (Photo by Robert Rogers); Right: Early summer

frostbite, hemorrhoids, boils, burns, and deeper or infected wounds. A tea of the inner bark is used for eyewash or ear cleansing. The tea is given for depression, or added to other herbs as part of a heart medicine.

FOLK USES

The inner bark of Tamarack is decocted to help bleeding of the lungs, or throat, and to soothe bleeding hemorrhoids. It will reduce excessive menstruation and is good for the liver and spleen when enlarged and hardened, combining well with Red Root. The warm, strained decoction is used in an eyecup for inflamed eyes, or dropped into the ear to relieve pain. The decoction is good to resolve gangrene or old skin ulcers, while a decoction of the wood ashes is better for healing burns and scalds. Fresh inner bark, containing galactic acid, is a healing poultice for wounds and frostbite. In cases of constipation, add wild licorice root and Calamus root to the inner bark and simmer slowly, one teaspoon of each to a pint of water for twenty minutes. Drink four ounces as needed. Tamarack cambium and bark has been found to possess high antioxidant activity, and may possess antidiabetic activity (Fraser et al. 2007).

PROPERTIES

Further work by Nan Shang et al. (2012) identified several compounds with antidiabetic activity. Rhapontigenin, previously identified, shows glitazon-like insulin sensitizing activity. A unique compound 23-oxo-3alpha-hydroxycycloart-24-en-26-oic acid showed strong adipogenesis activity at EC_{50} of 7.7uM. Another compound 13-epitorulosol also potentiated adipogenesis EC_{50} of 8.2uM. Like metformin and rosiglitazone, tamarack bark increases glucose uptake and adipogenesis, activates AMPK, uncouples mitochondrial function and improves ATP synthesis (Harbilas D et al. 2012). In a study by Owen et al. (1999) Tamarack extracts were found to exhibit the highest inhibition rate of xanthine oxidase at 86.33%. This is a good measure of success in treating gout. Phenolic and tannin contents are believed responsible for the activity.

Caution: The bark tea should not be used in combination with antibiotics.

Ledum groenlandicum (*Rhododendron groenlandicum*)
Labrador Tea

STOP 2

RUSSELL WILLIER

Willier calls this plant *maskihkohpakwa* or Muskeg Tea.

Leaves are made into a tea and drunk for pleasure or as a diuretic and for kidney problems. Occasionally it is used in combinations for internal problems such as bad blood and a stressed liver. It can also be used to lower blood sugar levels. The patient should drink a *maximum* of two cups once every three months.

ADDITIONAL CREE INFORMATION

The Northern Cree call the plant *maskihkohpakwa,* "plant of the muskeg," and make use of the dried leaves, even when gathered from under snow. The Woods Cree of Saskatchewan and nearby Hudson's Bay call it *kakiki-pak,* referring to the fact the leaves stay on the plant a long time. Eastern Cree call it *wesukipukosu,* meaning "bitter herbs." Other names include *mamîji'bagûk,* meaning, "hairy leaf," and *mamîzhi'bagûk,* "woolly leaf".

The leaves are combined with animal fats to treat burns. The leaves and flowers are made into tea for colds, combining with Calamus root for more severe conditions like whooping cough. The dried root powder is sprinkled on burns and skin ulcers until sticky and then replaced as needed.

FOLK USES

The Hudson's Bay Company imported the leaves into England as a beverage under the name *weesukapuka*. Stephen Leacock ([1920] 2009) wrote that the tea was "much used by the lower class of the Company's servants as tea, and by some is thought very pleasant. But the flower is by far the most delicate, and if gathered at the proper time, and carefully dried in the shade, will retain its flavor for many years and makes a far more pleasant beverage than the leaves." It has a mild, yet persistent diuretic effect that tones the kidneys, due to the drying nature of the herb. Decoctions of the leaves are very useful for itch and other skin disorders, especially when fever and skin eruptions are present. It can be used internally and externally. The aerial parts inhibit xanthine oxidase, associated with gout (Owen and Johns 1999). Work by McCutcheon et al. (1992) found the branches of Labrador Tea to be active against *E. coli, Bacillus subtilis,* and methicillin-resistant *S. aureus* or MRSA. Research in Quebec, led by Dufour et al. (2007), found that methanolic extracts of the Labrador Tea leaf possess anti-inflammatory and antioxidant properties. The twigs were also active against DLD-1 colon carcinoma and A-549 lung carcinoma cells, with ursolic acid identified as partly responsible for this cytotoxic effect. Further studies suggest it prevents the absorption of sugar in the small intestine due to alpha glucosidase inhibition. It appears to help in type-2 diabetes by either prior ingestion or taken with the meal, making this a possible great addition to alleviation of this pending epidemic (Baldea et al. 2010). Older texts suggested the herb contains arbutin and a toxic diterpene, acetyl andromedol. This is not true.

PROPERTIES

Research by Spoor et al. (2006) found that Labrador Tea (*R. groenlandicum*) extracts appear to possess insulinomimetic and glitazone-like activity.

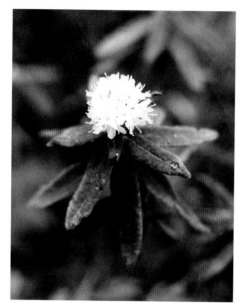 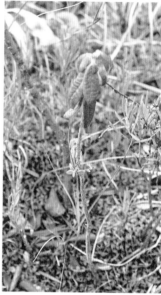

Left: Early summer (Photograph by research team); Right: Fall

Caution: The patient should drink a *maximum* of two cups of Labrador Tea once every three months according to Willier. It should not be used during pregnancy due to uterine stimulation.

Lonicera dioica
Twining Honeysuckle

STOP 11

RUSSELL WILLIER

Willier calls this plant *payipotakask* or Vine with a Hole in the Center.

It is used for heart problems and sugar diabetes. It can be cut into small chunks and used as a tobacco substitute.

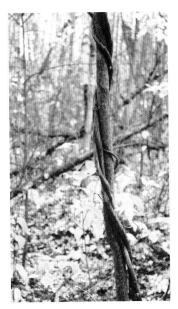 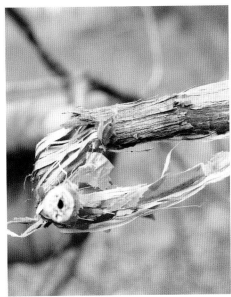

Fall

ADDITIONAL CREE INFORMATION

The Cree of Alberta call one of the species *owihkimakopakwa* or "nice-smelling leaves." The Cree of Saskatchewan call it Twining Honeysuckle *sipaminakasiwahtik* or *gaganonskiwaskwah*, meaning "long hair plant."

FOLK USES

The mature stems are soaked in water to make a hair rinse to help it grow. The inner bark is infused for use as a diuretic, and for flu symptoms. The stem is an ingredient in a mixture to treat blood clotting after childbirth and was used previously in attempts to cure venereal disease. The inner nodes are considered the most active part.

Studies in Turkey have shown that secologanin and various secoiridoids and glucosides from Honeysuckle possess hypotensive, sedative, antipyretic, antitussive, and tonic activity. Several of the Honeysuckles in our region contain these compounds in both the fruit and leaves, including this species (Rogers 2014).

Mentha canadensis or *M. arvensis* ssp. *borealis*
Wild Mint

STOP 2

RUSSELL WILLIER

Willier calls this plant *amiskowiyikaskwa* or Mint, Beaver Ears Leaves, or Beaver Roots.

Leaves are made into a tea and drunk for pleasure, to calm a fever, or to induce sleep. It is chewed as an aid to quit smoking, as well as to improve the smell and taste of combinations. It is found in semi-wet, churned-up grassy areas.

ADDITIONAL CREE INFORMATION

The Cree call it *amiskowiyikaskwa,* meaning "good tasting" or "delicious beaver plant," or *wiskask,* "pleasant tasting." The *Alberta Elders' Cree Dictionary* (LeClaire and Cardinal 1998) refers to mint as *ka tah-keyawepayesik.*

The leaves are infused for stomach disorders, coughs, colds, fever, menstrual cramps, to soothe teething pain, and for fatigue and insomnia. Wild Mint is used to treat high blood pressure and headaches, and is part of medicines for cancer and diabetes. Hot infusions help break a fever by inducing perspiration. Mint is used in traps as part of bait for lynx, or combined with beaver castor for red fox.

FOLK USES

The flowers can be applied directly to toothaches or inflamed gums, or inserted into the nostril to stop bleeding.

PROPERTIES

Luteolin, from the shoots, is an aldose reductase and xanthine oxidase inhibitor, suggesting use in complications associated with diabetes and gout. Ethanol extracts of *M. arvensis* appear to enhance the antibiotic activity of various drugs, such as gentamicin and chlorpromazine, against multi-drug-resistant *E. coli* (Coutinho et al.

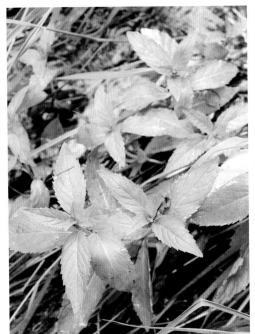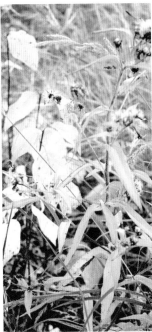

Left: Early summer; Right: Fall

2009). Wild Mint (*M. canadensis*) should be considered an ancient hybrid of *M. arvensis* x *M. longifolia,* according to work by Tucker and Chambers (2002).

Caution: Wild Mint has mild choleretic activity that may aggravate patients with gallstones. Patients suffering from GERD, or gastroesophageal reflux disease, should be very cautious with mint. Menthol opens the sphincter valve that connects the esophagus to the stomach and may aggravate an existing condition. Mint teas can bind up iron, so those treating anemia should take mint and iron a few hours apart. Do not take at the same time as antacids, H_2-receptor antagonists, or proton-pump inhibitors. Use with care around infants. Do not use during pregnancy, particularly during the first trimester, heavy menses, lactation, or cases with yin deficiency with heat, or deficient exterior patterns with sweating.

Mertensia paniculata
Lungwort, Tall Bluebells

STOP 1

RUSSELL WILLIER

Willier calls this plant *kasasiyoyakansiyohk* or King's Plant.

The root is used in combinations for breaking spells and as a good luck charm. The root also serves as a "protector" for the healer and in combinations for the heart. The root is mixed with tobacco for pipe ceremonies.

ADDITIONAL CREE
INFORMATION

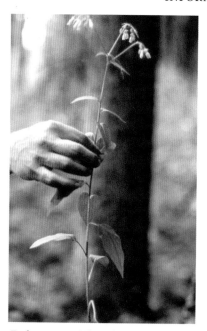

The Northern Cree call it Bluebells or *kasasiyoyakansiyohk*. Some Cree call it *ogu-malask*.

King's Plant is found in the boreal forest. The Cree named it a long time ago. It is the Bluebell of the boreal, and if ever the Cree nation had an item to barter with the rest of the world, this is it (Beresford-Kroeger 2010). The large leaves of nonflowering plants are gathered, sundried, and used with tobacco as a smoke.

FOLK USES

Early summer (Photo by research team)

Lungwort makes an acceptable oyster-flavored potherb, but it is a little hairy for salads. Dried leaves can be saved for addition to herbal tea mixtures, especially when treating the lungs. The roots make a very good edible bush food, steamed, boiled, or roasted like parsnips. This herb is stimulating to the respiratory system, much like its close relatives Borage and Comfrey. Congestion and deep-seated emotional issues can be resolved with the use of both the herb and the flower essence. The astringent qualities of this herb make it effective in relieving diarrhea and hemorrhoids. The leaves make useful poultices for external cuts and wounds, as well as over the lung region for respiratory problems. The cool, moist nature of the leaves alleviates hot, dry, inflamed conditions of the lungs, as well as the skin (Rogers 2014).

Nuphar variegatum
Yellow Pond Lily

STOP 5

RUSSELL WILLIER

Willier calls this plant *waskwatamoh* or Water Lily.

The root is chewed for ulcers, heartburn, or indigestion. It is also chewed or made into a tea to treat coughing up blood from prescriptions. It is used in combinations for skin problems and for circulation.

ADDITIONAL CREE INFORMATION

The Cree of Alberta use several names, including *pwakumosikum, askayamo, oskotamo, waskwatamoh, waskutamo, osk-itipak,* or *waskiti-pak,* meaning "leaf."

The Woods Cree of Saskatchewan use the dried roots for winter food. The fresh roots can be sliced and fried in fat or boiled, but consumption should be limited, especially because it tastes like swamp! The flower buds can be cooked and eaten, or pickled like capers in vinegar. The Woods Cree combine Water Lily, Calamus, and Cow Parsnip root as a salve for painful joints, limbs, swellings, and headaches. As a poultice, these three are used for treating worms that infect the flesh of humans or horses. The rhizomes are cut into thin rounds and dried. Then they are made into a tea for arthritis, or used to bathe the affected area. When poulticed or grated, the fresh root can be applied to boils, diabetic skin ulcers, sore backs and legs, or infected wounds.

Compound decoctions are used to help women recover from child-birth, are given during birthing to assist delivery, or are part of heart or cough medicines.

FOLK USES

The dried rhizome can be chewed raw, or dried and then cooked later in winter. The fresh root, particularly as a tincture, is useful for vaginal, uterine, or ovarian irritation in the female, and prostate or penile irritation in the male. For testicular or scrotal hydrocele, combine with Red Root. A douche of the root tea, or a sitz bath with a weak decoction, may be helpful. The root cools and shrinks hot, inflamed, and painful conditions, but is not for dull, congested, subacute conditions that require stimulation. The root can be used as a poultice for an acute state of rheumatoid arthritis or inflamed, swollen joints, such as gout and pseudo-gout.

PROPERTIES

The Yellow Pond Lily roots contain a complex mixture of quino-lizidine alkaloids that have a broad range of antibacterial, antifungal, and antiyeast activity. They have estrogenic activity, and exhibit prostaglandin synthetase inhibition. Ethanol extracts show activity against gram-positive bacteria. Some of the alkaloids may be sedative,

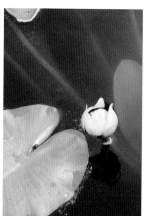 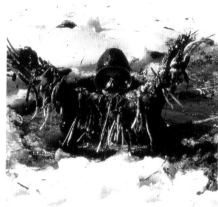

Left: Summer; Right: Collecting roots in winter

hypotensive, and antispasmodic in activity. Nupharine has antispasmodic and blood-pressure-lowering activity similar to that of atropine and papaverine. Mice studies show it inhibits lung tumor formation. Desoxynupharidine is tonic in nature and can elevate blood pressure. A sugar compound present in the fresh root of *N. variegatum* exhibits activity against *Staphylococcus aureus* and *Proteus vulgaris*. Nupharin A is active against *S. aureus* and *Saccharomyces cerevisiae* (Nishizawa et al. 1990).

Caution: Do not use in constipation or deficient conditions. It has a mild immune-depressing effect. Stop use if the cold sensation in the body is exaggerated.

Parmelia sulcata
Waxpaper Lichen
—
STOP 8

RUSSELL WILLIER

Willier calls this plant *waskwiya* or Moss.

This moss found on the Diamond Willow is chewed and put on the gums (for one-half minute) of babies with pain from teething. The sap is used for sugar diabetes. It is an excellent fire starter when dry.

FOLK USES

Also known as Powdered Shield Lichen, this is a common branch lichen on dead Spruce branches throughout the north. Rufous hummingbirds use it to decorate and hide their nests. In Italy, various species of *Parmelia* are used as a cholagogue. Because it contains salazinic acid, it can also be used for dyeing wool.

PROPERTIES

The lichen acids, including salazinic and lobaric, are antiseptic. Salazinic acid is an alpha-glucosidase inhibitor, meaning that it decreases the amount of sugar transported from the intestine to blood plasma. Therefore, it helps low blood sugar in diabetes (Verma et al. 2012).

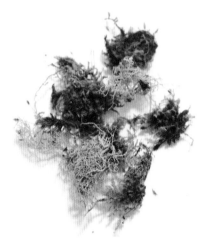

Summer (Photo supplied by Shutterstock)

The lichen shows activity against various bacteria and fungi, including *Aeromonas hydrophila, Bacillus cereus, B. subtilis, Listeria monocytogenes, Proteus vulgaris, Yersinia enterocolitica, Staphylococcus aureus, Streptococcus faecalis, Candida albicans, C. glabrata, Aspergillus fumigatus, A. niger,* and *Penicillium notatum* (Candan et al. 2007; Rankovic et al. 2007).

Petasites sagittatus
Arrow-leaved Coltsfoot

STOP 11

RUSSELL WILLIER

Willier calls this plant *miyokatayinipiya* or Frog Leaves.

The leaves are chewed, then used on cuts and slivers. Bad infections are wrapped in the underside of a leaf. It is also used for blistered feet and athlete's foot.

ADDITIONAL CREE INFORMATION

The Saskatchewan Cree call the flower *wapathaman*, and the leaves *mosotawakayipak*, meaning "moose ear leaf," or *yuwskiyhtiypuk*, meaning "soft leaves." The Alberta Cree call Arrow-leaved Coltsfoot *piskehtepask*, meaning "separate leaf," in reference to the leaf and flower coming at separate times. The flower can bloom up to one month prior to the appearance of leaves. In northern Alberta, the Cree know it as *puskwa* or commonly refer to it as "wolverine's foot" or "owl's blanket" due to its insulating value.

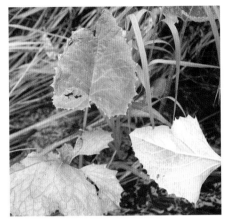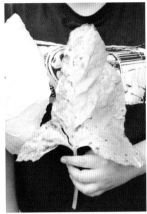

Left: Early summer; Right: Fall

The furry inside of the leaves is gathered by birds to line their nests. The roots are soaked in hot water to make a tea, taken internally for tuberculosis, sore throat, stomach ulcers, and such. It appears to stop the internal bleeding associated with these conditions.

FOLK USES

Native people use Coltsfoot for coughs, colds, and other bronchial complaints. The leaves are rolled into balls, dried and burned, and used as a salt substitute. The leaves are dried and later soaked in warm water and applied to open sores and ulcers. The dried roots are grated and applied to boils or running sores. The roots are best harvested before flowering, but are sometimes difficult to find. Coltsfoot as warm tea will assist the body by inducing sweat and relieving chest pain. It stimulates the lungs to expel phlegm, and it eases asthmatic wheezing with its antispasmodic action. Combined with Sundew, it is useful in whooping cough, bronchitis, asthma, and other difficulties. It combines well with fresh Nettle leaf for hay fever and allergic rhinitis. It stimulates the immune system and fights infections in the bladder, skin, and lungs. Coltsfoot root decoctions are helpful for external ulcers and chronically weeping wounds.

PROPERTIES

Petasin, a sesquiterpene of petasol and angelic acid, is the most active antispasmodic component. It suppresses a protein in the blood that plays a role in triggering bronchial spasms, according to Kahlee Keane (2012), also known as Root Woman, an accomplished Saskatchewan herbalist.

Caution: Due to the plant energetics, do not combine Coltsfoot with Goldthread or Oregon Grape root. Avoid in individuals with phase 2 liver detoxification problems. One study found hepatic toxicity when taken at two hundred times the normal daily internal dose.

Picea glauca
White Spruce
STOP 4

RUSSELL WILLIER

Willier calls this plant *siyihtah* or White Spruce.

A small tree is stood up near the house to protect a large area, such as a farm, from curses. It is changed once a year.

ADDITIONAL CREE INFORMATION

The Northern Cree call this *sihtipikow*. When speaking generally about White Spruce, the Cree will call it *siyihtah*.

The Cree use it for waterproofing baskets, canoes, and the like. The gum is pounded together with charcoal to make glue that sticks when hot to set arrowheads and spear points before binding. It is smeared on burnt pine torches for greater efficacy, and to waterproof strips of hide for snares and snowshoes. It is a good medicine for infected wounds and stomachaches. When boiled with Spruce cones, water, and lard, the mixture turns pink and when cooled makes an ointment the Cree call *pikim*. This is used to draw infection from cysts or to soothe various skin rashes, including chicken pox. The small, immature cones are chewed by the Cree for sore throats, whereas the tender young tips are peeled and eaten to prevent shortness of breath, or held in the mouth to treat hypertension and heart problems. The wood is harvested for construction purposes, due to its flexibility and relative strength. Both the Cree and the Chipewyan use Spruce for traps, snares, meat drying racks, snowshoes, hide-stretching frames, or the frame of Spruce bark canoes. The inner bark is scraped out and chewed for colds, or dried for later use. The outer bark is stripped off large trees in the spring when the sap is running, and used to make smokehouses for drying fish.

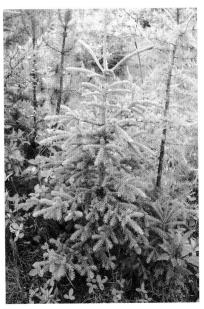

Summer

FOLK USES

The Spruce gum or pitch collects on trees in a form reminiscent of brittle tears. It is collected and burned in the same manner as frankincense. This is preferred to plastic or canvas, due to the constant inside temperature that can be maintained. The rotten wood is used to smoke tanned hides. White Spruce needles show cytoprotection against both glucose toxicity and glucose deprivation in work by Harbilas et al. (2009).

Picea mariana
Black Spruce
___
STOP 1

RUSSELL WILLIER

Willier calls this plant *minahyik* or Black Spruce.
  Cones are used for stomach problems.

ADDITIONAL CREE INFORMATION

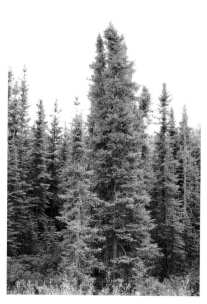

Summer

Black Spruce is called *minahyik* or sometimes *wapasiht.* Black Spruce is known as *itinatik,* the "people tree," or *napakasihta,* and is sometimes called Swamp Spruce, *maskekosihta.*

The Cree use the strong and pliable roots for weaving baskets and setting snares. It will sometimes yield knotless, straight-grained wood that, cut green and split 90 degrees to the grain, will yield very thin plies that can be woven into waterproof baskets for cooking. It is often twisted, but experienced eyes can spot the straight ones. Native people, in the past, would limb a growing tree that was straight, so that their children or grandchildren would have knot-free wood with which to work. The small green cones of Black Spruce provide a red dye for porcupine quills.

FOLK USES

Snow blindness results in a whitening of the affected pupil. If allowed to develop unhindered, sight will be lost. A balsam of young Black Spruce tops is made by cutting upper shoots of the sapling and then bending and splitting in two. These are left by the fireside and after the resinous liquid is heated out, the eyeball is gently coated with the balsam using a bird quill. Rogers does not recommend this treatment (Rogers 2014). Hot water extracts of Black Spruce bark show benefit against psoriatic keratinocytes, suggestive of psoriasis relief, in a study of numerous native Quebec trees by García-Pérez et al. (2010).

PROPERTIES

Black Spruce extracts contain an insulin sensitizer that exerts its effect through PPAR activation. PPAR agonists, such as rosiglitazone, increase the sensitivity of muscle and adipose tissue to insulin (Spoor et al. 2006). Recent work from the group looking at seven traditional Quebec Cree plants for diabetes found that the activity is analogous to that of metformin, and it is not an insulin signaling pathway. Rather, insulin sensitivity is AMP activated by the protein kinase pathway (Martineau, Adeyiwola-Spoor, et al. 2010).

Pinus banksiana
Jack Pine

STOP 1

RUSSELL WILLIER

Willier calls this plant *askatikos* or Jack Pine.

New buds are used in combinations for a variety of ailments. Bark from a young tree is used in a combination for removing curses. The inner bark is used in the sweat lodge.

ADDITIONAL CREE INFORMATION

The Chipewyan call Jack Pine *gani,* whereas some Cree call it *oskahtak,* and Lodgepole Pine is *oskahcakosak. Oskayi* means "new."

The Cree make a strong thread from the fibrous roots called *watape,* used to sew together sheets of Birch bark for canoes or cooking vessels. They also melt the pitch to fumigate sickrooms.

FOLK USES

Jack Pine roots can be fifty to sixty feet long, with a consistent circumference. These are split, coil wrapped, and placed in the water to more easily remove the bark. The long pine needles come in handy for sewing jobs that don't require as much strength, or are used to make baskets. Some Native tribes believe evil spirits live in Jack Pine, causing infertility in women and animals.

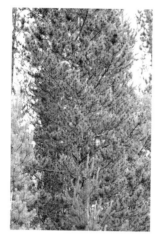
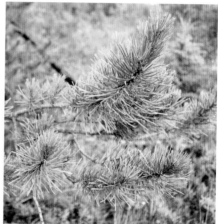

Summer

Pine needles contain isocupressic acid. This has been found to cause abortions, metabolizing into imbricatolic, agathic, dihydroagathic, and tetrahydroagathic acids. The cones of Jack Pine display strong antioxidant activity (Fraser et al. 2007).

Polygala senega
Seneca Snake Root, Milkwort, Seneca Root

STOP 5

RUSSELL WILLIER

Willier calls this plant *miyinsiyikîysa* or Bead Berry.

The whole herb is used in combinations for heart problems and as a blood purifier. Tops and flowers are mixed with Red Osier Dogwood as a tobacco substitute.

ADDITIONAL CREE INFORMATION

The Alberta Cree call it *miyinsiyikîysa*. The Wood Cree of Saskatchewan know it as *winsikis*.

The Alberta Cree chew the aromatic root for toothache, as well as sore mouth and throat. They use it for various heart problems related to aging, such as irregular heartbeat, coughs, and nervousness. The Cree carry the root on long journeys to ensure health and safety.

FOLK USES

Seneca Root is an official drug in Germany and France, where it is highly valued for its stimulating and expectorant properties. This is useful in chronic bronchitis, croup, asthma, pneumonia, whooping cough, and other congestive lung conditions. It was official in the US Pharmacopeia from

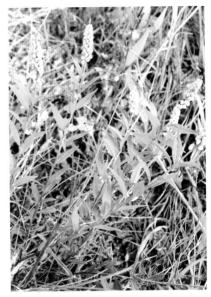

Summer

1820 to 1936 and in the US National Formulary from 1936 until 1960. In Canada, the root is used in about a dozen drug products for coughs.

Seneca Root acts as a local stimulant in congested, sore throats and is an excellent gargle for either laryngitis or pharyngitis. Both polygalic acid and senegin are irritants to the gastrointestinal mucosa, and cause a reflex secretion of mucus in the bronchioles.

Phillips (1879) wrote: "In the advanced stages of pneumonia, when there is much prostration and the cough dry, harsh and painful, with a sense of oppression across the chest, this medicine promotes expectoration and relieves other distressing symptoms." In the bronchitis of old people and especially when complicated with emphysema, Seneca often acts beneficially (Rogers 2014).

Caution: Avoid Seneca use during pregnancy or for patients with a history of gastritis or IBD. Overdosing will induce vomiting, diarrhea, and CNS depression. Avoid if allergic to salicylic acid, or while taking blood thinners. Be cautious with stomach ulcers. Seneca Root will exaggerate a feverish state or inflammation, and should not be used at this stage.

Populus balsamifera
Black Poplar, Balsam Poplar

STOP 9

RUSSELL WILLIER

Willier calls this plant *mayîmiyitos* or Black Poplar.

Fresh roots of a newly uprooted tree are used for acne, and also in combinations for purifying the blood. Buds are used for healing wounds.

ADDITIONAL CREE INFORMATION

The Cree call it Ugly Poplar, *mathamitos,* or *mayîmiyitos,* meaning "rough looking." The punk from the inner bark is called *apustam* and is used for the ceremonial lighting of pipes. The Cree call the leaf buds *osimisk.*

Buds are sometimes placed in hot bathwater and allowed to steep until a layer of extract forms on the surface. The patient with eczema or psoriasis then enters the bath. It is messy but effective, as water and resins do not mix. Teething babies have the buds rubbed directly on their gums, while buds can also be placed in the nostril to stop nosebleeds. The dried inner bark of Balsam Poplar makes a suitable soap, as do the Aspen leaves and branches when boiled in water. The ashes are used for cleaning buckskin or washing hair, by soaking them in water overnight, and straining off the upper part.

FOLK USES

The new spring buds are collected and gently simmered in vegetable oil, 1:5 ratio of weight to volume. This oil is a good anti-inflammatory for joint pain, chest congestion, and obstinate constipation when taken internally. The buds are dried and ground into a powder that is mixed with oil as a salve, or cooked with animal fat over low heat. This is used on a baby's umbilical cord for healing. The bark makes waterproof shingles that resemble adobe tiles. The Cottonwood fluff gives a pleasant smell to blankets when used as insulation. The Hudson's Bay Company mixed the inner bark of Balsam Poplar with tallow to make soap. The larger Balsam Poplars and Cottonwoods can be tapped like Birch and the sap drunk fresh. It is used to treat diabetes and high blood pressure. Likewise, the buds and Aspen bark (see *Populus tremuloides* below) are decocted for diabetes. The bark and sap are boiled together to make a tea given to children with asthma, or it can be boiled down to a gooey consistency to serve as wood glue, tightly holding its bond under stress and resisting cracking from dryness.

PROPERTIES

Balsam Poplar buds show a very low LC_{50} rate against neuroblastoma cells, in work by Mazzio and Soliman (2009) that looked at 374 natural products for antitumor activity. The inner bark of Balsam Poplar shows antagonistic activity against PPAR gamma, suggesting use in obesity and other metabolic conditions (Martineau, Hervé, et al. 2010). Recent work found that ethanol extracts of Balsam Poplar bark mitigate the development of obesity and insulin sensitivity in diet-induced mice. Inhibition of adipocyte differentiation, decreased liver inflammation, and increases in hepatic fatty acid oxidation were found (Harbilas et al. 2013). The extract decreased glycemia and improved insulin sensitivity by diminishing insulin levels and the leptin/adiponectin ratio.

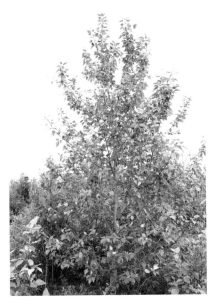 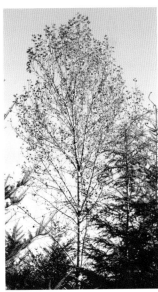

Left: Summer; Right: Fall

Populus tremuloides
Trembling Aspen, Aspen Poplar

STOP 2

RUSSELL WILLIER

Willier calls this plant *miyotohs* or White Poplar.

A two-inch-long twig about one inch wide can be boiled for diarrhea or stomach cramps.

The green bark is chewed for food poisoning. Bark is used in combinations and as a "representative" of the healer in the spiritual world.

ADDITIONAL CREE INFORMATION

The Cree call Aspen Poplar *meitos, miyotohs, mistik,* or *wapisk-mitos,* meaning "white tree."

The Cree shred the bark, especially in the spring, and made a liquid extract for coughs. One elder of the Assiniboine had this to say about the sweet-tasting cambium layer of Aspen Poplar: "We always call it ice cream trees, because they're sweet and they're juicy. Let's go and eat ice cream juice, we'd say." It is said to taste like honeydew melon. Women steep the roots of both Black Poplar and White Poplar together as a tea to stop bleeding during pregnancy and prevent premature labor. Aspen leaves (*mitosinipiah*) are chewed and applied to bee or wasp stings, mosquito bites, and cuts.

FOLK USES

The inner bark is a nourishing food, either boiled or ground into flour. This flour can be used for food, or mixed with the sun-dried leaves of *kinnickinnick* and tobacco as a more mellow smoke. The inner bark can be cut into spaghetti-like strips and boiled. The white powder on the south-facing side of Aspen bark is mixed with fat and applied as a sunblock, deodorant, and antiperspirant. It is scraped off and applied to cuts and deep wounds to coagulate and stop bleeding, can be applied directly to bee stings to reduce swelling, or can be used as a substitute for talcum powder. This white yeast is reflective and protective for the Poplar as well, preventing the premature flow of sap from late winter or early spring sunlight. Mors Kochanski says that some Natives mixed the white powder with the vitreous humor of eyeballs of animals as body paint or for artifacts (personal communication). The yeast is gathered and added to flour and water to produce a type of sourdough starter. It takes a few days to start working and then can be added to dough for bannock and such. The bud resin, extracted with alcohol, can be used sparingly as a kidney tonic. Dribbling and irritating urination, especially atonic bladder, calls for Aspen Poplar bark, combining well with Bearberry leaf. According to Matthew Wood (2009, 278), "Poplar is beneficial in conditions where there is fear, hyperadrenalism, hyperthyroidism, and overactivity of the sympathetic branch.... It reduces fever and heat, and establishes groundedness and strength, in people who are nervous." He has used the tincture successfully in cases of asthma associated with hyperthyroidism.

PROPERTIES

Populin relaxes the nervous system, and relieves headaches due to liver or stomach acidity and gas. Populin is licorice tasting, and glycosides influence stomach and digestive tract health. Populin, like salicin, converts to salicylic acid in the system. Poplar helps where there is lack of urine flow, due to prostate or kidney inflammation. This may be due to the zinc lignans or the flavonoids in both the bark and leaves of Aspen Poplar.

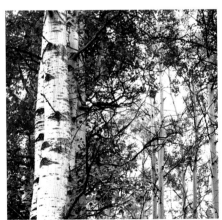 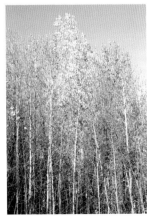

Left: Summer; Right: Fall

Prunus pensylvanica
Pin Cherry

STOP 9

RUSSELL WILLIER

Willier calls this plant *nipinimina* or Summer Berry (Summer Willow). He calls the tree *nipinanatik.*

It is used in combinations for removing a curse.

ADDITIONAL CREE INFORMATION

The Cree call the berry *pusawemin,* or Tart Berry, and mixed them with bear grease and powdered meat to make pemmican. Another Cree name for the tree is *nipinanatik.*

The Cree use the inner-bark decoction to treat sore eyes, a common affliction due to summer sun, snow blindness in winter, and inadequate smoke ventilation. The flexible, yet strong new growth is used for tipi pins, food skewers, arrows, bows, pipe stems, medicine pipe tripods, bow drills, and even toothpicks. The wood does not absorb water, and makes for good firewood after a rain. The dried bark is smoked for headaches and head congestion. The fresh bark of Pin Cherry makes a very acceptable wilderness adhesive tape—simply peel and tape in place. This same flexible bark was used to wrap and strengthen the joints of harpoons, spears, bows, and arrows. The bark was smeared with Pine or Spruce pitch and bound with sinew or Dogbane fiber, making a waterproof bond.

PROPERTIES

Matthew Wood (2009, 286) says, "In addition, it contains cyanogens, which break down into hydrocyanic acid. This stops the Krebs cycle, which is the body's mechanism for producing energy. Thus, cyanogens cut down heat production at the cellular level. This is why too much cyanide can kill a person. Fortunately, the amount of cyanide in a small dose of wild cherry bark is only enough to cool. The cyanogens and flavonoids work together to sedate and cool the organism."

Caution: Pin Cherry and Choke Cherry bark are contraindicated in pregnancy, due to their teratogenic potential and the cyanogenic glycoside prunasin. If gathering the bark yourself, wait until past midsummer. The content of prussic acid will be lessened—avoiding problems of depressed respiration. Prunasin is highest

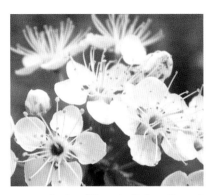

Spring (Photo by Robert Rogers)

in bark that is green and is actively photosynthesizing. However, the easiest time to collect the inner bark is in the spring, when the bark slips away easily from the wood. It's best to wait until there are berries. Peel off the outer bark, and then peel away the inner bark in long strips for drying. Other sources suggest that HCN is highest in bark collected in the fall, about 0.15 percent, whereas spring bark is only one-third of that, at 0.05 percent. After drying, store carefully, as it loses medicinal properties quickly when exposed to light or oxygen. It's best to make a tincture as soon as it is dried, for an optimal product.

The largest concentration of cyanide is in the large succulent leaves on vigorous shoots. Livestock will sometimes eat this if a pasture is poor. Cattle and horses can die, whereas deer, moose, and elk eat the winter twigs and leaves with no problem. Be careful—it can produce cyanide poisoning, with the resultant cellular hypoxia (you can die). If you suspect poisoning, induce vomiting or gastric lavage, and afterward antidote with a sodium nitrate IV, followed by a 25 percent solution of thiosulfate. If the patient is unconscious, the acidosis is corrected, shock is treated, oxygen is administered, and a cyanide antidote such as amyl is given. If the patient has had a seizure, use a diazepam IV; in methemoglobinemia, use an emergency exchange transfusion. The most important antidote is cobalt EDTA, also known as Kelocyanor®. Due to its own toxicity, sodium thiosulfate is a good partner to support the body's own detoxification system. In slight poisoning, the latter may be useful on its own (Rogers 2014).

Prunus virginiana
Choke Cherry, Circle Berry

STOP 9

RUSSELL WILLIER

Willier calls this plant *tokwayîminana* or Choke Cherry (Circle Berry). It is used in combinations for removing a curse.

ADDITIONAL CREE INFORMATION

The Cree call it *takwayîminana* or "berry that is crushed." Various plains Natives call the time during fruiting "black cherry moon."

The dried berries are used in pemmican for winter. A tea from the dried leaves, stems, bark, and root is used for treating colds, fevers, and pneumonia, or to clear the throat of singers and speakers, as it loosens phlegm. The bark is used to treat diarrhea, or a decoction is strained and cooled then used as a douche. The Cree use green wood skewers to both attach and flavor meat over a fire. The bark is decocted for diarrhea and dysentery, sometimes with the addition of Marsh Valerian and Sweet Cicely Root.

FOLK USES

Frejnagel and Zdunczyk (2008) found the polyphenols of Choke Cherry prevent damage from oxidized fats in the diet. A traditional preparation is to crush the berries between two stones, and form into cakes to dry. You can then warm them up in a pan with lard and sugar. Traditionally, Choke Cherries are stored in small animal skins, with Wild Mint stuffed in the leg openings to keep the berries from falling out, and yet allow enough air in so they do not mold. Choke Cherry bark has a toning and stimulating effect on the digestion and a sedative action on the nervous system. It cools stomach and liver heat and nervous tension experienced as stomachache. One of its primary functions is to relieve irritation of the mucous membranes—be it the urinary, digestive, or respiratory system. The dry root or inner bark is infused or gently simmered for stomach inflammation like acidosis or gastritis, or for treating diarrhea. This is probably due to astringent tannins in the bark. During recovery from pneumonia, pleurisy, and even acute hepatitis, Choke Cherry bark soothes, without overstimulating.

PROPERTIES

Choke Cherry bark is a peripheral antitussive. Irritated tissue near or below the larynx is relieved by antitussive herbs, whereas coughs up higher are best resolved with demulcents.

Choke Cherry fruit inhibits aldose reductase, and reduces the expression of both IL-1 beta and COX-2. It causes a strong inhibition of inflammation and has the ability to reduce the development of microvascular complications of diabetes, including retinopathy and neuropathy (Kraft et al. 2008).

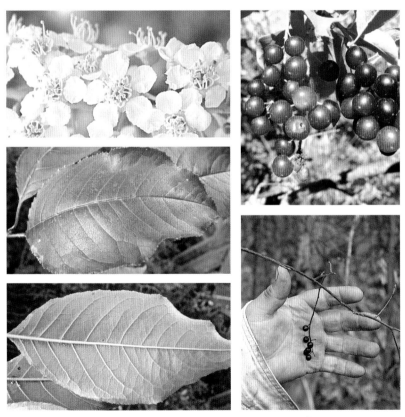

Clockwise: Spring, Summer, Fall, Summer, Summer
(All photos by Robert Rogers except bottom right)

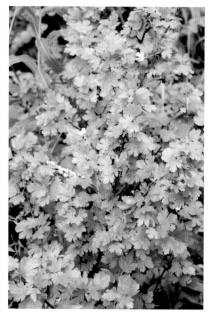

Summer

Ribes oxyacanthoides
Northern Gooseberry

STOP 8

RUSSELL WILLIER

Willier calls this plant *sapominahk* or See-through Berry.

The root is used for eye problems and also in combinations for the heart. The berries are eaten.

ADDITIONAL CREE INFORMATION

The Cree know this plant as *sapominahk,* meaning "transparent berry" or "bitter berry." The root is boiled for delayed menstruation, whereas the stem is steeped as an infusion for stopping excessive bleeding after childbirth or used as part of a combination for sickness after giving birth.

FOLK USES

The unripe Gooseberry has been shown to prevent degeneration of cells in studies from Russia. Gooseberry leaf makes a good infusion to lessen the menstrual pain of young women, and to help prevent the formation of kidney stones. The leaf tea is used to treat chronic diarrhea, and dysentery. Gooseberry juice can help relieve painful skin conditions like Rosenbach's disease or erysipelas, either alone as a wash, or combined with Elderberry juice (Rogers 2014).

Rosa woodsii
Wild Rose

STOP 8

RUSSELL WILLIER

Willier calls this plant *okiniyi* or Wild Rose.

One red and one white piece of stem are boiled together to make a tea for breaking a severe curse. The tea can also be drunk for pleasure.

ADDITIONAL CREE INFORMATION

The Alberta Cree call it *kaminakuse*, thorn plant, or the longer *okamina-kasiwahtik*, while the Woods Cree of Saskatchewan use the shorter name *okiniyi*. The Cree call the rose gall *wiposi*.

The Cree peel and boil the inner bark of Prickly Rose stem or root, and apply the cool liquid to sore eyes.

FOLK USES

The bitter, red root decoctions are boiled for an hour, to treat bad coughs. The taproot of Wild Rose can go down more than twenty feet, making it a drought-resistant plant. Four branches are decocted and drunk to relieve excessive menstruation, whereas the root is used for

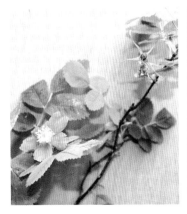 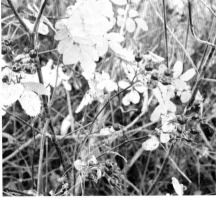

Left: Early summer; Right: Rose hips in fall

correcting an irregular menstrual cycle (Rogers 2000). The galls, produced by the cynipid wasp, *Rhodites rosae,* are burned and crushed in Traditional Chinese Medicine and dusted on burns. Closer to home, the Pawnee did the same thing—thousands of miles and an ocean apart.

PROPERTIES

Kashiwada et al. (1998) found that oleanolic, alphitolic, and pomolic acids from Wild Rose (*R. woodsii*) leaves inhibited HIV-1 replication in acutely infected H9 cells. Oleanolic acid had a therapeutic index of 12.8, while pomolic was 16.6.

Rubus arcticus
Arctic Raspberry, Dwarf Raspberry

STOP 8

RUSSELL WILLIER

Willier calls this plant *oskisikomina* or Eye Berry.
The root is sometimes used for the heart.

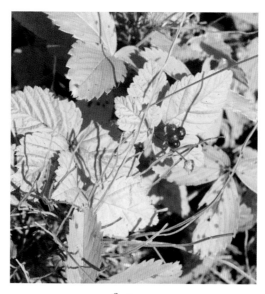

Summer

ADDITIONAL CREE INFORMATION

The Cree know it as *oskisikomin*, meaning "eye berry." The Alberta Cree call Raspberry *ayiskanahk*, meaning "soft berry," and like numerous tribes, used decoctions of the root or leaf for various female problems involving childbirth. The Saskatchewan Cree call it *athoskan*, or *anoskana*, meaning "broad berry."

The young stems can be peeled and eaten, or dried and made into a decoction to treat fevers. The roots are boiled and the cooled decoction used for eyedrops in snow blindness. The unpeeled root and stems are made into a tea for children's diarrhea, stomach pain, teething, and to help slow menstrual bleeding.

FOLK USES

Dwarf Raspberry has bright-pink, narrow-petal flowers on ankle-high plants with no prickles. The fruit is tasty, but is only found singular. The Dena'ina called them frog's cloudberry, or frog's berry.

Rubus idaeus or *R. strigosus*
Raspberry
—
STOP 8

RUSSELL WILLIER

Willier calls this plant *ayiskanahk* or Raspberry.

Roots are used in combinations for removing a curse, as well as for high blood pressure, blood sugar stabilization, and purifying the blood. The berries are eaten.

FOLK USES

A survey by McFarlin et al. (1999) of American Certified Nurse-Midwives in the late 1990s found that 63 percent recommended Raspberry leaf tea as a uterine tonic. A randomized, double-blind, placebo-controlled study of 192 women by Simpson et al. (2001) suggests Raspberry leaf may shorten labor in pregnant women and reduce the need for medical intervention. The second stage of labor was shortened by nine minutes, and the rate of forceps delivery was only 19.3 percent, compared to more than 30 percent for a control group. A controlled, retrospective observational study of 108 pregnant women suggests the herb may shorten labor, reduce the likelihood of preterm and postterm labor, and reduce the need for medical intervention. Three cups daily was the most popular dosage, with the majority beginning at around thirty weeks (Parsons et al. 1999).

PROPERTIES

Like many herbs, Raspberry leaf has an amphoteric effect on uterine muscle, causing both contraction and relaxation of myometrial muscle, as needed.

Caution: Be very careful to use either very fresh leaves, or completely dried leaves. The drying process can produce various toxins that disappear with complete drying. The best leaves are from the tops of the first-year growth. The fruit should be avoided in urinary difficulty associated with yin deficiency with heat.

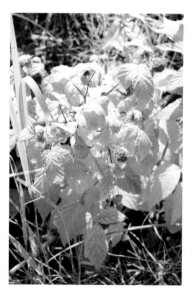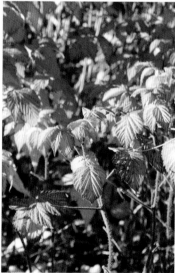

Left: Summer, Right: Fall

Salix bebbiana
Diamond Willow

STOP 10

RUSSELL WILLIER

Willier calls this plant *nêpisiyiwaskwôto* or Diamond Willow.

Saplings are used for framing a sweat lodge. The bark is sometimes used in combinations.

ADDITIONAL CREE INFORMATION

The Cree call Diamond Willow *nipis.*

It is valued for the inner bark, which is edible and can be eaten raw or shredded and cooked like pasta, even ground into a powder for making bread. The catkin fluff is used to line baby cradles. The root bark is mixed with kidney fat to heal sores and dandruff of the scalp. The Woods Cree steep the inner bark of Pussy Willow, *acimosihkansak*, for treating diarrhea, and like other Natives, use the tannins to cure animal hides.

FOLK USES

Some botanists believe fungi cause lesions on Diamond Willow; others disagree. Bebb's or Diamond Willow has been used to make baseball or cricket bats, and at one time, the bast fiber, or inner bark, was used to make fish nets and lines in the north, where Stinging Nettle or Dogbane was not available. Some say it is the best! Root decoctions of Bebb's Willow are used for problems of fatigue associated with circulatory disturbance. Salicin from the inner bark is broken down by healthy intestinal bacteria and then conjugated with enzymes in the liver to salicylic acid. This compound possesses anti-inflammatory and analgesic effect, without blood thinning or stomach irritation. Dioscorides, in the first century AD, suggested catkin tea for sexual overstimulation, or whenever the urogenital system is inflamed and overexcited. Oribasius around 360 AD suggested fern root with willow leaves be taken after coitus for contraception. Aëtius in the sixth century suggested a mixture of boiled Willow bark and honey for contraception. Constantine

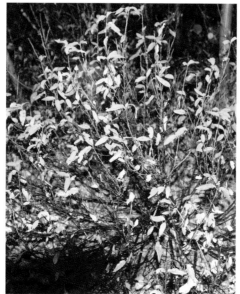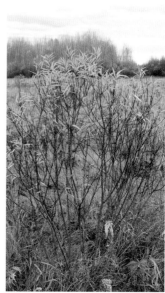

Left: Early summer; Right: Fall

the African in 1085 advised using the juice of willow leaves so that a woman will not conceive.

Today, the catkin and Pussy Willow water are used for the same purpose in cases of genital discharges and sexual excess that exhausts the body. Products imported from Lebanon are called "Pussy Willow Water." The fact that the catkins contain estriol explains a lot of its traditional usage. The distillate of catkins is known as Arq e Bedmushk and is used in Unani medicine for nervousness and palpitations of the heart associated with stress (Rogers 2014). Some individuals sensitive to tinnitus may find that Willow bark causes aggravation. There is a human case report of contraindication associated with genetic predisposition to glucose-6-phosphate dehydrogenase deficiency. Autopsy reports of the great composer Ludwig van Beethoven suggest a possible link between his chronic use of powdered Willow bark and development of renal papillary necrosis, according to Schwarz (1993).

Sarracenia purpurea
Pitcher Plant

—

STOP 8

RUSSELL WILLIER

Willier calls this plant *ayikitas* or Frog Pants.

It is used in combinations for menstrual problems, coughing, back problems due to the kidneys, and to increase urine flow.

ADDITIONAL CREE INFORMATION

The Woods Cree of Saskatchewan know the plant as *athikacas,* meaning "little frog pants." The Cree know the plant as Frog's Legs, and used it for those who were very sick. In the *Alberta Elders' Cree Dictionary* (LeClaire and Cardinal 1998), the Pitcher Plant is known as *askihkosihk kohpikihcikesihk.*

Cree healers use it for respiratory and heart ailments, often in combinations. The root was decocted and given to a woman to prevent sickness after childbirth, and combined with other plants in decoction to expel the afterbirth.

FOLK USES

The first recorded use of this plant was by the Native people of Canada. Smallpox, carried from Europe, caused a widespread epidemic among the previously unexposed Native population. With no natural immunity, the death rate was alarmingly high. The leaves of this plant exhibit marked antidiabetic activity in vitro (Muhammad et al. 2012). The compounds hyperoside and morroniside exhibit a protective effect against diabetic neuropathy (Harris et al. 2012). A proprietary liquid extract of *S. purpurea* powdered root, called Sarapin, has been locally injected by physicians treating neuralgia. Manufacturers of the product list painful syndromes relieved by Sarapin as sciatic pain, intercostal neuralgia, alcoholic neuritis, occipital neuralgia, brachial plexus neuralgia, meralgia (thigh) paraesthetica, lumbar neuralgia, and trigeminal neuralgia. These are pinched or trapped nerves, reminiscent of the entrapment strategy of Pitcher Plant.

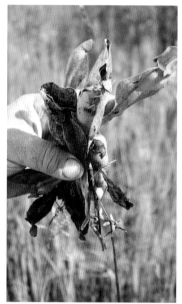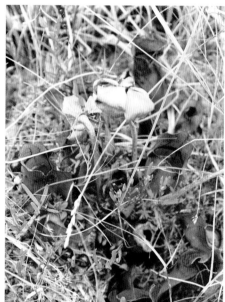

Left: Summer; Right: Fall

PROPERTIES

Like Sundew and Stinging Nettle, the fresh plant contains histamine, which is anti-inflammatory, a vasodilator, and a bronchoconstrictor. It can be used topically to relieve chilblains, and internally to promote gastric pepsin secretion. Spoor et al. (2006) examined eight indigenous plants of Quebec used traditionally for diabetic-like symptoms. Pitcher Plant (*S. purpurea*) extracts appear to possess insulinomimetic activity, as supported by a rapid and insulin-independent effect on glucose uptake in muscle and fat cells. The effect was quantitatively greater than that of 400 micromol/L of metformin. It showed protection under both cytotoxic conditions tested. Pitcher Plant is protected by CITES (Convention on International Trade in Endangered Species) of Wild Fauna and Flora, to save it from extinction.

Shepherdia canadensis
Buffalo Berry, Soapberry
————
STOP 8

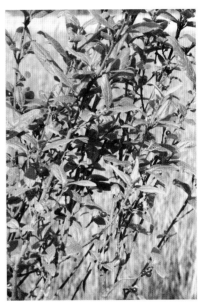

Summer

RUSSELL WILLIER

Willier calls this plant *kinipi-knipsi* or Snake Willow.

It is used for skin problems and eruptions.

ADDITIONAL CREE INFORMATION

The Woods Cree of Saskatche-wan know Soapberry as *kinip-ikominanahtik,* meaning Snake Berry Tree. It is also called *kinip-ikomina,* or Snake Berry Plant.

They use plant decoctions externally for aching limbs and arthritis. The stem is considered important in the treatment of venereal disease, whereas the inner bark is infused as a reliable laxative. The berries contain saponins that relieve skin problems. The most recent twigs are used in decoction to prevent miscarriage. A decoction of the fresh, split-peeled roots and split twigs was given to reduce fever in babies, or used as a rub or rinse for sore mouths. The root has been add-ed to heart medicines, in an unspecified manner. Twigs and roots are strongly laxative and have been used traditionally for chronic coughs and tuberculosis.

FOLK USES

Mors Kochanski says that the winter tips of Buffalo Berry are an endor-phin inducer, and used by Natives to fend off hunger pains and oth-er discomforts of winter living (personal communication). Harmine, harmane, and harmaline alkaloids may be responsible, in part, due to their MAO inhibition (antidepressant effect). He has observed that the branch buds appear to grow in winter, which is quite unusual. It is one of two ingredients in a "Northern Ayahuasca" traditionally used for shamanic vision quests (Rogers 2014).

Caution: Buffalo Berry is a mercury accumulator, so be careful in polluted regions.

Smilacina racemosa (*Maianthemum racemosum*)
False Solomon's Seal
——
STOP 2

RUSSELL WILLIER

Willier calls this plant *kawawkanaht* or Backbone Root.

The root is used in combinations for headaches, as well as for kidney and back problems.

ADDITIONAL CREE INFORMATION

The Cree of Alberta call it *kawawkanaht,* meaning "it's his (or her) back." The root looks like the disks of a human spine.

FOLK USES

Numerous Native tribes use the root tea to regulate menstruation, and the leaf tea as a contraceptive. The root contains diosgenin, a precursor to progesterone. The leaves are infused for chest colds, and the ends are soaked and used to wet and soften the hair and keep away dandruff. Solomon's Seal and False Solomon's Seal roots are used for a variety of problems affecting the joints, bones, tendons, and ligaments. Matthew Wood (1997, 399) puts it well: "I have seen so many cases of stretched, loose or tight tendons cured by Solomon's Seal that I can hardly count them—probably over a hundred … [It] is suited to conditions where the ligaments and tendons are loose or tight, it adjusts the tension on the connective tissue to the right level. This prevents injuries and corrects old traumas. It also feeds and lubricates the ligaments, tendons, muscles and attachments, making the muscular and skeletal system stronger and more harmonious in its actions." Repetitive injury syn-

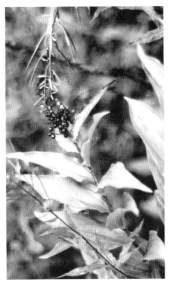 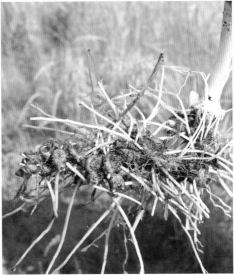

Left: Summer (Photo by research team); Right: Root in fall

dromes such as tennis elbow, jogger's knee, carpal tunnel, and such respond to both internal and external applications (Rogers 2014).

Solidago canadensis
Canadian Goldenrod

STOP 3

RUSSELL WILLIER

Willier calls this plant *ohsawicêyipêyihk* or Goldenrod.
 Used in combinations.

ADDITIONAL CREE INFORMATION

Some Cree call Canadian Goldenrod *chachamos kakew,* meaning "it makes one sneeze," whereas the Northern Cree call it *ewaposawak nephehkan.*
 Tea prepared from the leaves and flowers has been used traditionally for sensations of paralysis. The young flower heads make an effective thickening agent for bush soups.

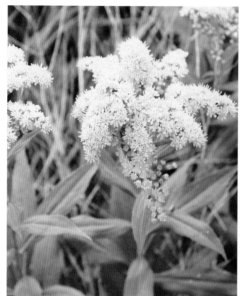 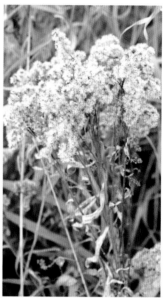

Left: Early summer; Right: Fall

FOLK USES

The pollen is heavy and does not cause allergic respiratory distress, for which it is blamed. Two main organs are affected by Goldenrod: the kidneys and the upper respiratory system. To both these areas, a drying, cooling, and restorative property is imparted due to the bitter and pungent nature of the plant. Water retention is decreased so that acute urinary obstructions are relieved. Swollen ankles and puffy eyelids are a key symptom to the use of this herb. Both excess urea and cholesterol are removed, along with gravel and small stones. The herb is a reliable aquaretic, increasing urine release and reducing inflammation due to infection or irritation from stones and gravel. Work by McCune and Johns (2002) at McGill University found Canadian Goldenrod extracts more powerful in antioxidant activity than green tea or ascorbic acid.

Caution: Do not use in cold, deficient conditions.

Sorbus americana or *S. decora*
American Mountain Ash

STOP 12

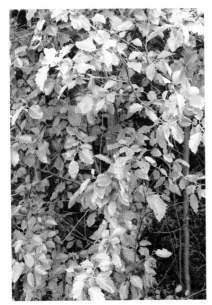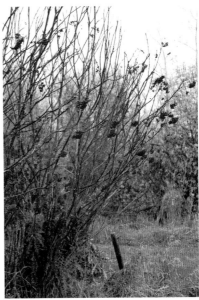

Left: Early summer; Right: Fall

RUSSELL WILLIER

Willier calls this plant *asiniyociyipiyk* or Mountain Ash.

The root is used for the heart, liver, kidney, and blood, and as a tea. The bark can be used in combinations for removing curses.

ADDITIONAL CREE INFORMATION

To the Northern Cree it is sometimes called the same as Red Willow, *atospiy*. To the Bush Cree, a Red Mountain Ash branch is known as *comiaykwachoowass-oot*. Other Cree names for the tree are *maskominanatik* and *esniywachi-wahtik*. The Cree of southern Saskatchewan call it Western Mountain Ash, Bear Berry Tree, or *maskwaminanahtik*. The Woods Cree call it *maskocisk*.

147

The Cree of northern Alberta harvest the roots, then dry and grind them as a coffee substitute. They use the branch bark for pleurisy and inflammatory disease, including internal bleeding. The Saskatchewan Cree decoct the bark for bones, while branches are decocted for the heart, and unspecified parts for treating cancer. Some Natives boil the branches and steam themselves to relieve headaches and sore chests. The Cree of the Wabasca, Alberta, area use the root as part of diabetic and cancer treatments. The Manitoba Cree use inner-bark decoctions without berries to treat backaches and rheumatism. The leaves are decocted for flu. The inner bark is chewed or boiled for constipation.

FOLK USES

Decoctions of fruit are used for heart health, helping to reduce blood pressure, fibrillation, and angina pain. This is due to the hexanoic form of parasorbic acid, which is a potent beta-adrenergic blocker, according to Diana Beresford-Kroeger (2010). Extracts of bark show anti-hyperglycemic and insulin-sensitizing activity *in vivo*. Vianna (2011).

Sphagnum fuscum
Peat Moss, Sphagnum Peat Moss
STOP 8

RUSSELL WILLIER

Willier calls this plant *maskwoskwa* or Peat Moss.
It is used on cuts and infected areas, and for baby diapers.

ADDITIONAL CREE INFORMATION

The Cree of Saskatchewan and Alberta call it *askiyah* and use it for wiping, as paper towels are used today, and traditionally for cleaning babies of mucus and blood after birth. The Cree call Green Peat Moss *maskwoskwa*.

FOLK USES

Native people mix the green Sphagnum Moss with animal fats to treat cuts. It is the first disposable diaper material, because of its absorbency and disinfecting properties. Sphagnum Moss is capable of holding twenty times its weight in water. Sphagnol, extracted from Peat Moss, is used for hemorrhoids and for various skin problems such as psoriasis, eczema, and acne. Work by Painter (2003) found sphagnum dressings three to four times more absorbent than cotton dressings.

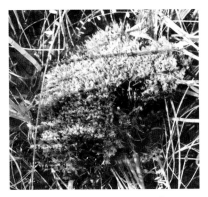

Summer

PROPERTIES

The herb pectins react chemically against various proteins, and immobilize whole bacterial cells, as well as enzymes, exotoxins, and lysins secreted by various pathogens. Peat Moss is used in several commercial feminine sanitary napkins.

Taraxacum officinale
Dandelion

—

STOP 13

RUSSELL WILLIER

Willier calls this plant *osawciyipiykwa* or Dandelion.

The roots are used in combinations for purifying the blood.

ADDITIONAL CREE INFORMATION

Meyoskamewuskos or "spring plant," as known to the Cree, is used for laxative (roots) and diuretic (leaves) action. It is called *osawapikones* in the *Alberta Elders' Cree Dictionary* (LeClaire and Cardinal 1998).

FOLK USES

Dandelion leaf is one of our best organic sources of potassium, making the leaves one of our safest, most balanced diuretics. It helps remove excess water, uric acid, and sodium, thereby reducing hypertension. It helps tone anabolic stress conditions, and by increasing potassium, it reduces muscle spasms and nighttime leg cramping. It is especially useful in treating elevated systolic blood pressure in the elderly. This is due not only to potassium, but also to vitamin C, luteolin, and caffeic acid in the leaves that all contribute diuretic activity. A small study of seventeen patients showed significant diuretic activity from ethanol extracts of the leaf (Clare et al. 2009). Nine compounds with diuretic effect have been identified. Dandelion root clears obstructions from the liver, spleen, and gallbladder and helps balance high or low blood sugar states related to the pancreas. By assisting the liver, without irritation, it can help clear up many skin problems. An easy way to think of the actions of Dandelion root is that it opens what is blocked, cools what is irritated, and drains what is soggy (Rogers 2014).

Caution: Do not use in cases of closure of the biliary ducts, gallbladder congestion, or ileitis. It will promote biliary secretion that can severely exaggerate symptoms—be sure of the condition. This is based on theoretical views of choleretic action, and not empirical or clinical observation. Dandelion root extracts may also cause overproduction of stomach acids, leading to irritation of gastritis or stomach ulcers. Dandelion root use may exaggerate lithium toxicity, and should be avoided when taking quinolone-type antibiotics due to the possibility of diminishing their effectiveness or worsening side effects.

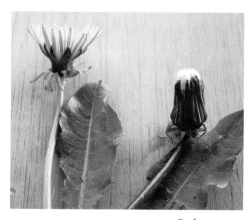

Early summer

Trifolium pratense
Red Clover
———
STOP 5

RUSSELL WILLIER

Willier calls this plant *mostosmetisowihn* or Clover.

It is made into a tea for chest and lung problems. It also helps pimples and to purify the blood.

ADDITIONAL CREE INFORMATION

The Cree had no medicinal uses for the newly introduced plant, but named it *maskosiya* or *moostos mechewin,* meaning "cattle food."

FOLK USES

The flowers have a long, folkloric history for skin problems, including acne, eczema, and psoriasis. It has been called the "Queen of the Blood Purifiers," in reference to its alterative action on kidney, liver, and bowel function.

PROPERTIES

The leaves contain isoflavones that mimic phytoestrogenic activity, binding to receptor sites and easing undesired symptoms in menopausal women (Rogers 2014).

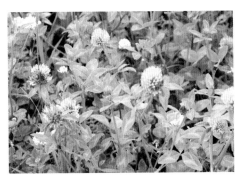 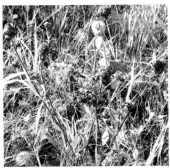

Left: Early summer; Right: Fall

Typha latifolia
Cattail

—

STOP 8

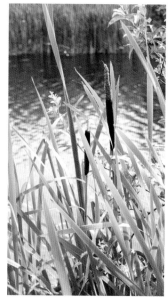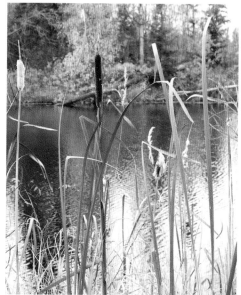

Left: Summer; Right: Fall

RUSSELL WILLIER

Willier calls this plant *ohtawaskwa* or Ocean Plant.

The fluff is mixed with grease to make a poultice for first-, second-, and third-degree burns. It will also help prevent infection.

ADDITIONAL CREE INFORMATION

The Cree call it "plant of the middle of the water," *osawîyowaskwa*, or *watotahuk*.

The down from the mature female head is used as diaper padding by the Cree, who also call it *otawask*, meaning "water edge plant." The flower spike, *pasihkan*, is burned to ash and applied to a new infant's navel. The down is applied to burns and scalds as a dressing. It is combined with tallow or animal fat as a sort of chewing gum. The pollen and tallow are combined to condition hair damaged by sun and wind.

FOLK USES

Cattails can be gathered when up to a foot tall in the spring and cut off at ground level. Within two weeks, another shoot will appear. The taste when raw is like cucumber, and when boiled or steamed, they become more slimy, like okra. The Dene of northern Canada brew the lesser cattail tea for dysuria, or inability to pass urine. The burned spike ash is smeared on skin rashes in young children from moss diapers. The fruit polysaccharides initiate keratinocyte formation, suggesting skin-healing properties (Gescher and Deters 2011).

Urtica dioica
Stinging Nettle
STOP 5

RUSSELL WILLIER

Willier calls this plant *masan* or Thistle.

The top or root is boiled to make a tea for increasing urine flow.

ADDITIONAL CREE INFORMATION

The Cree call it *masan* or *masanak,* meaning "itchy weed." The plant fiber is gathered in fall when the plant begins to die. It is retted, like hemp, before the fiber is extracted. The Cree use leaf decoctions to stop the blood flow or hemorrhage after childbirth. The root can be boiled and the steam inhaled for asthma. Leaf decoctions are used as a wash for acne, and internally for diarrhea or intestinal worms. The stems only are decocted for urinary difficulty in men.

FOLK USES

Various First Nations peoples of the prairies use Stinging Nettle. The Nitinaht of British Columbia made Nettle fiber until the 1970s. The fiber of Stinging Nettle has high tensile strength, fineness, excellent spinning quality, and cell walls that are unlignified. The fibers have low

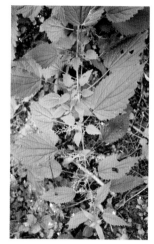 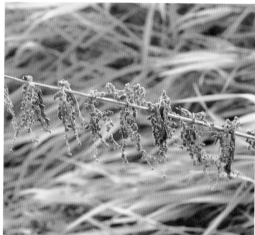

Left: Early summer; Right: Fall

specific gravity and high strength, with a good elasticity or stress rating. The fresh juice stimulates kidney activity and is a valuable alterative or blood cleanser. In human clinical trials (Belaiche and Lievoux 1991), the fresh juice produced marked diuretic activity in patients with myocardial and chronic venous insufficiency, and showed hemostatic activity. When Nettle leaf is used to bring down blood pressure, the passage of sand and gravel in the urine may be considered a good sign. Roschek et al. (2009) found the extract of benefit for allergic rhinitis due to inhibition of COX-1 and COX-2, inhibition of mast cell tryptase, and various other key receptors and enzymes, including agonism and antagonism against the histamine 1 receptor. Hematopoietic Prostaglandin D_2 synthase inhibition, which blocks this primary pro-inflammatory mediator, was also noted. Stinging Nettle root extracts were studied by French researchers on sixty-seven men with varying degrees of prostate enlargement, and showed positive nighttime urination control in about two-thirds of individuals. At least thirty clinical trials have been conducted on the root for both BPH and prostatitis, ranging in size from only 20 to 5,492 participants (Rogers 2014). Cold Nettle leaf tea alleviates the itch associated with Hodgkin's disease.

PROPERTIES

Nettle hairs contain small amounts of histamine and leukotrienes. Contrary to popular belief, they do not contain formic acid. A chemical cocktail of histamine, acetylcholine, and serotonin, as well as other compounds, accounts for the stinging sensation.

Caution: Stinging Nettle leaf reduces the body's production of interleukin-6, which regulates the immune system, and should be avoided by those coming down with or in the early stages of influenza. The plant contains 5-hydroxytryptamine, which is an isolated uterine stimulant, emmenagogue, and abortifacient. Fresh plant extracts can induce uterine excitation, or contractions. Some authors suggest the root should be used with caution with antihypertensive, diabetes, CNS depressive, and diuretic medications (Rogers 2014).

Valeriana dioica
Northern Valerian, Marsh Valerian

STOP 1

RUSSELL WILLIER

Willier calls this plant *apiscakowaskos* or Small Arrow.

The root is used to purify one's hands as well as in combinations for good luck charms and for breaking curses. The tops can be used as a tobacco substitute.

ADDITIONAL CREE INFORMATION

The Cree of Alberta call Marsh or Northern Valerian *maskihkewahtik,* meaning "a plant with medicinal value." The Woods Cree of Saskatchewan call it *apis-cisakweskwos,* meaning "small strong smell."

Various Native tribes rub their traps with the root scent to attract bigger cats like mountain lion, cougar, and lynx. The Cree chew the root to prepare a poultice for earache. They use a poultice externally to treat seizures in young children, a wise choice considering the antispasmodic effect of Valerian. The leaves are boiled for forty-five minutes until the water turns green. This is given to children who have lost weight. The stems and leaves are boiled to treat sore, aching bodies, colds, chills, and congestion, and to help clear air passages. Two cups of the dried leaf decoction are given to pregnant women to prevent miscarriage or ease labor pains. The dried leaves are mixed with beaver fat and applied to facial rashes. A root decoction from a Valerian plant that has not flowered is considered a powerful tonic for someone who feels bad. Ethanol extracts are used as antidandruff rinses. A piece of the root can be held in the mouth or chewed for severe heart trouble. The Saskatchewan Cree chew the root, then place it in aching ears. The root is chewed and rubbed on the head and temples for headaches, as well as externally on babies with seizure activity. The root is used to treat pneumonia and is added to smoking mixtures for colds. The dried leaves are a pleasant smoke. In cases of swollen glands in children, a hot root fomentation is applied to the affected area. The plants without flowers are considered stronger and are known as male, whereas the female plants with flowers are used but are not as prized. The leaf is said to work faster and better. The root is used for heart complaints. It is added to love medicine, or *sakihitowask,* that attracts the affections of another. This is considered a bad medicine or curse. The whole, dried plant is crushed, passed through Diamond Willow Fungus smoke, and carried in a pouch over the heart as a good luck charm. A controlled clinical trial on eighty-two chronic heart disease patients, with angina pain, showed Valerian root reduced symptoms by 87 percent (Yang and Wang 1994).

PROPERTIES

By inhibiting the breakdown of GABA, the increased neural activity preceding epileptic seizure may be moderated or prevented. Water extracts possess anticonvulsant activity mediated through activation of the adenosine system (Rezvani et al. 2010).

Caution: Valerian should be used for several weeks and then off for a week. In excess, it can produce mild dependence and create the same symptoms it initially treated. In extreme cases, excessive use can cause paralysis and cardiac problems. Valerian root is also constipating for some individuals, and can pose a problem if consumed long term without laxative support. Acute toxicity is rare; consumption of twenty times the recommended dosage results in significant side effects, but no toxicity. Brinker (2001) says that forty or more 470 milligram capsules will create toxicity that can be treated with activated charcoal. An eighteen-year-old woman ingested forty to fifty tablets in a suicide attempt. All her mild symptoms resolved in twenty-four hours, suggesting that at twenty times the therapeutic dose, Valerian appears benign (Willey et al. 1995). In tincture form, Valerian should never be used in excess conditions, or in full heat, fevers, or inflammation. The exception is the use in acute conditions like migraine or epilepsy. In addition, it should not be taken with any sleep-inducing drugs or barbiturates as it may potentiate their action. It may, however, enhance the action of Hops, Poppy, Skullcap, or Vervain. It has no dangerous synergistic activity with alcohol, as suggested in some books.

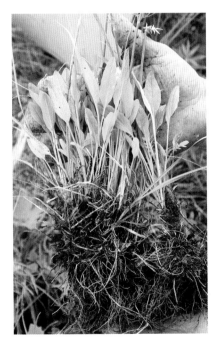 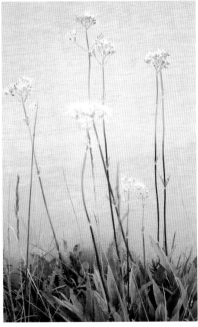

Left: Early summer; Right: Summer

Viburnum opulus (*V. opulus* var. *americanum*)
High Bush Cranberry, Cramp Bark

STOP 9

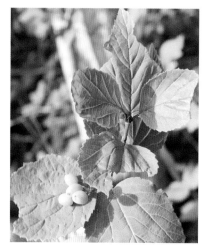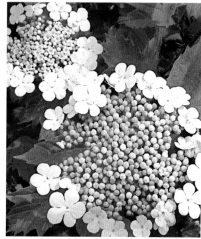

Left: Early summer; Right: Spring (Photos by Robert Rogers)

RUSSELL WILLIER

Willier calls this plant *nêpiminana* or High Bush Cranberry.

It is used in combinations to remove a curse. The berries are a good food source.

ADDITIONAL CREE INFORMATION

The Cree call High Bush Cranberry *nipiminan,* meaning "summer berries," whereas *mongsoa-meena* or *mosomina,* meaning "moose berry," is the low bush variety. The former was corrupted by traders and voyageurs into Pembina—hence the name of the river in Alberta. In some books you will read that Pembina or Pimbina is derived from the Cree *nipiminan,* meaning "berry growing by the water." An 1853 journal from the Red River suggests the name comes from *anepeminan,* with *nepen* meaning summer, and *minan,* berry. I believe the latter is correct.

Bark tea is used by the Cree as a diuretic, and to prevent postpartum infections in new mothers after childbirth. The bark tea is used for insomnia.

FOLK USES

The inner bark of Cramp Bark contains the properties leading to its name. Collected in May, the vibrant-green inner bark possesses antispasmodic and nervine properties useful for many parts of the body. Cramp Bark relaxes the uterus and relieves menstrual pain, combining well with Valerian root when the pain is severe. Cramp Bark combines sour and acrid properties that help reduce both heat and tension. These qualities of moving, relaxing, and cooling make it most useful in menstrual pain and excessive menstrual bleeding. It relieves the pain of endometriosis and orchitis. Threatened miscarriage in the third trimester with rhythmic cramping and little or no spotting is stopped. In habitual miscarriage, the herb can be taken one to two teaspoons daily well into the second trimester if needed. In threatened miscarriage, one teaspoon every hour is taken until the crisis has passed. Later, the herb is given prior to labor, preparing the uterus for the vigorous activity coming. And finally, it is given to reduce the severity of afterpains and uterine spasms. The herb nourishes the heart, quiets the spirit, and clears heat from the heart, making it a useful addition for insomnia, anxiety, and depression (Rogers 2014). High Bush Cranberry fruit inhibits aldose reductase, improves glucose uptake, reduces inflammation, and modulates energy expenditure. This suggests a role for the berries in preventing diabetic microvascular complications such as retinopathy, and perhaps in insulin resistance and metabolic syndrome (Kraft et al. 2008).

PROPERTIES

Scopoletin is involved in the secretion of serotonin, helping to reduce anxiety and depression.

Caution: Women and children, including teenagers, who are allergic to aspirin (Reye's syndrome) should avoid *Viburnum* ssp. In some individuals it may aggravate tinnitus, or ringing in the ears. It may lower blood pressure, so be cautious. Avoid use with blood thinners.

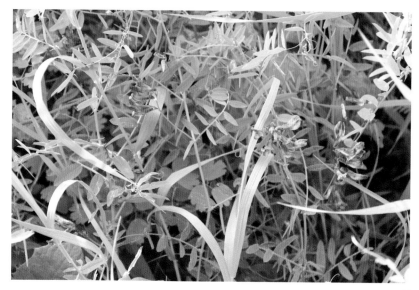

Fall

Vicia cracca
Purple Vetch, Tufted Vetch

STOP 13

RUSSELL WILLIER

Willier calls this plant *kiyiminkiyowask* or Climbing Vine.

The roots are used in combinations for the heart, as well as for stomach cramps.

FOLK USES

Tufted Vetch is an introduced perennial with purplish-blue flowers and a weak, sprawling stem. It was originally brought to North America centuries ago as a fodder or a green manure that since then has escaped and flourished. The unripe seeds look like small peas, but contain traces of hydrocyanic acid that is removed by cooking. The ripe seeds can also be sprouted.

PROPERTIES

Tufted Vetch contains pyrimidine derivatives that cause photosensitivity illness. Two patents exist for *V. cracca:* one is for its lectins' potential as an antiretroviral drug. The lectin is blood type A specific. It accumulates cyanamide. This compound is an alcohol-deterrent drug in Canada. The hair-loss drug Minoxidil and various anthelmintic drugs are derived from cyanamide (Rogers 2014).

The other uses affinity adsorbents for isolating lectins. One-chain lectins are specific to blood type A. The plant contains nineteen phenolic compounds, nine flavonoids, as well as quercetin, kaempferol, apigenin, and diosmetin. The latter compound may degrade to diosmin after intestinal bacterial action. Diosmin has been found useful in treatment of chronic venous insufficiency by prolonging the vasoconstricting effect of norepinephrine on the vein walls, increasing tone and reducing hypertension. It also reduces the release of prostaglandins, in turn reducing inflammation. Tufted Vetch (*V. cracca*) leaves in a water extract show activity against mycobacteria.

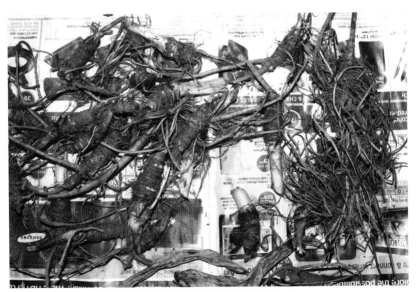

Drying herbs that have been cleaned and washed

Cleaning and Storing

After plants have been picked, they should be cleaned of extraneous materials and thoroughly washed within a day or two, after which the plants are dried for several days to prevent mold and rotting. They can then be stored in plastic bags or glass jars in a cool, dry place where insects and mice cannot cause damage.

Samples of each of the most commonly used plants are kept in the healer's medicine bundle with his ceremonial objects. The medicine bundle is used for traveling to ceremonies or to visit patients.

Willier ties herbs belonging to combinations together and keeps these little packets in his medicine bundle, as well as a written list of the herbs included in each combination, in case something happens to him and the bundle is passed on to someone who might not know what the herbs are for.

Most healers use other things besides plants, such as animal and bird parts and minerals. Willier uses products from bear, horse, dog, beaver, goose, and skunk. Minerals representing the different colors and directions are also used: yellow, red, and black clays, as well as coal and salt.

Part III

The Efficacy of Native Medicine

Efficacy is difficult to define because whether a medicine or a treatment works depends partly upon one's expectations. The expectations of a patient may differ from those of his or her family, and the expectations of a Native healer may differ from those of a medical researcher. A patient may be happy if he or she feels better, whereas a medical researcher might argue that simply making one feel better can be achieved with a placebo. A medical researcher may not be convinced of efficacy unless a pathogen has been removed, there is significant improvement in a diseased organ, or a large-scale, double-blind study provides statistical proof.

When I first talked to Russell Willier about the possibility of documenting his healing practices, he felt that if we could demonstrate the efficacy of Native medicine according to Western medical standards, young Native people would be encouraged to have faith in their own cultural traditions, and Western medical scientists would be encouraged to take Native medicine seriously and to cooperate with Native healers to improve the health of all Canadians. It was impossible to investigate the efficacy of Native medicine with the gold standard of Western medicine, a double-blind study, for several reasons. First, Russell considered it unethical to provide some patients with the hope of recovery while they were really only receiving sugar pills. Second, Native healing practices are not compatible with handling a large number of people, as Native healing requires rather intensive interaction with a patient over a period of time, and Native ceremonies such as a sweat lodge ceremony are limited to around a dozen people. Finally, all medicines must be administered in a proper ritual context in which spiritual and psychological factors are encouraged to interact with medicinal ingredients in the medicine itself. The best we could do was to elect a before-and-after procedure in

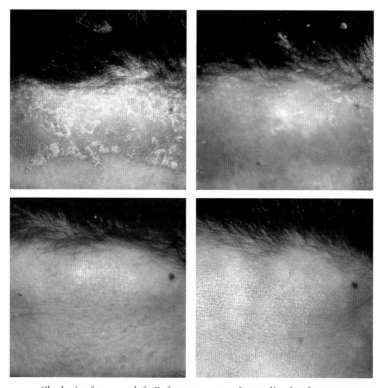

Clockwise from top left: Before treatment; Immediately after treatment;
Two months after treatment; Seven months after treatment.

which a patient's condition was photographed before treatment, immediately after treatment, and several months later. This type of "case study" approach is valuable in that it provides an in-depth record of a patient's condition and produces hard evidence in the form of photographs that can be supplemented with interviews with patients, as well as medical assessments using high-tech equipment and procedures by Western medical personnel.

Even our before-and-after procedure, however, was considered radical at the time in the Native community, in that Native healers were not in the practice of allowing their treatment procedures and ceremonies to be photographed. The research design was also criticized by other anthropologists who frequently argued that Native medicine should

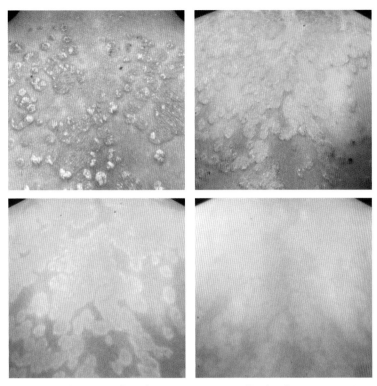

Clockwise from top left: Before treatment; Immediately after treatment; Two
months after treatment; Seven months after treatment
(Photos taken by a medical photographer)

be judged on its own terms and that imposing Western scientific standards for measuring efficacy is an example of cultural imperialism.
From the point of view of Russell and the researchers, however, this
attitude was patronizing because it set a different standard for measuring efficacy, even though the healer himself wanted to be assessed by
Western standards.

The situation was complicated even further by some Western medical personnel who were upset that we would be using research money to study "witchcraft." Despite all the problems and controversy, we
decided to proceed with the Psoriasis Research Project, in which non-
Native patients with psoriasis were treated at an Edmonton inner-city
clinic and in sweat lodge ceremonies. As described in the Preface, six of

ten patients experienced significant improvement, one of whom was completely cured of psoriasis on his hands.

Teenagers Treated at the Reserve

Despite the fact that doctors at the clinic judged the experiment to be a success, Russell was disappointed, as he felt there should have been better results. He subsequently treated several patients at his reserve, including two teenagers whose conditions were extremely severe. Both patients were photographed before treatment, immediately after treatment, two months later, and seven months after treatment, using the case study approach described above. In both cases, results were dramatic. The young man had stopped attending high school because he was so badly disfigured. After being treated by Russell Willier, his psoriasis cleared up and he was able to complete school.

The young woman had a similar experience. Immediately after treatment, while visiting relatives with her parents in Calgary, she developed a high fever and her skin began to peel all over her body. Her parents immediately took her to the hospital, where she remained for a couple of days until the fever returned to normal, after which she and

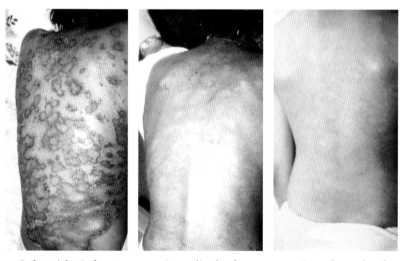

Left to right: Before treatment; Immediately after treatment; Several months after treatment (Photos taken by her father)

her parents returned to Toronto. Researchers maintained contact with the young man for two years and with the young woman for five years. During those periods, the psoriasis reappeared in very limited areas a couple of times but quickly disappeared with an additional treatment.

Personal Experience

In 1987 David Young's wife, Michiko Young, came down with a high fever and diarrhea. She was taken to the emergency room at the University of Alberta Hospital, where she was eventually placed in isolation because her fever remained high for ten days, she was in and out of a coma, and she was diagnosed with something like Legionnaires' disease. On the tenth day, I was informed by the doctors that they could not bring the fever down or stop the dehydration and that I should be prepared for the worst. At that point, Michiko's weight had dropped to around eighty pounds and her hair was coming out.

That evening I phoned Russell Willier to ask for help. Russell said that he had had a vision instructing him to pick certain herbs because someone would be calling for help. He said he would be at our house early the next morning. After he arrived, we sat at the dining room table cutting up the herbs and making tea, which was placed in glass jugs. We took the medicine to the hospital, where we informed the staff that Russell was a relative. As soon as we entered Michiko's room, Russell purified the room and persuaded Michiko to drink a little of the tea through a straw. By four in the afternoon, her fever had begun to drop, to the surprise of the doctors. When I told Russell about her diarrhea, we went immediately in search of some green bark of a young Trembling Aspen tree. When we returned to the hospital, Russell masticated the bark and put it in Michiko's mouth. The diarrhea stopped immediately. Russell returned home to collect roots to stimulate Michiko's appetite. After using these roots, Michiko sat up in bed and began to eat anything available, as she was constantly hungry. Michiko stayed in the hospital for three weeks, during which time she began the long, slow process of recovery. She had to relearn many things, as she could not even add two and two after coming out of the coma. Eventually, however, she made a full recovery and today is in excellent health.

The Mouse Woman of Gabriola

After I reestablished contact with Russell in 2010, Russell visited our home on Gabriola. While there, he visited a nearby petroglyph of the Mouse Woman, carved in a large vertical rock in a forest setting. The Mouse Woman is a Grandmother spirit important to West Coast peoples. In addition to helping rectify injustices to young people, the Mouse Woman also has healing powers. Russell found that the Mouse Woman provided "spontaneous healing" for his badly damaged leg due to hitting a moose with his truck three years earlier. After that, Russell returned with various patients to be treated by the Mouse Woman. During treatment, Russell offered tobacco and said prayers while patients leaned up against the Mouse Woman. Patients reported feeling heat and something like an electric current coming from the rock. All patients treated in this way experienced partial or full recovery from a variety of ailments, including arthritis.

Deborah Gray

While praying in front of the Mouse Woman, a branch from a nearby Arbutus tree fell at Russell's feet. He took this as a sign that he was to incorporate this plant into his medicinal repertoire. He took Arbutus bark with him when he returned home. One night he had a vision in which he was instructed on how to combine the Arbutus bark with other local herbs and which ailments to treat with this new combination. He subsequently used the combination successfully for the treatment of liver problems, heart problems, sugar diabetes, and high blood pressure.

Deborah Gray was a patient treated for liver problems that were so severe that her doctors had sent her home from the hospital to die, saying that her liver disease was so advanced they could be of no help. Deborah's partner phoned Russell, asking for help. Russell began treating her with the new combination, and within four weeks her liver had returned to normal. I had the privilege of interviewing Deborah and her partner while conducting fieldwork with Russell in October 2011.

How Do We Explain Such Results?

It is widely accepted that chronic diseases have a large emotional or spiritual component, often associated with stress. Because chronic diseases make up the bulk of ailments for which people visit a doctor or an emergency room, they are an important aspect of health care in any country and an important cause of health care costs that threaten to escalate out of control. Traditional therapies, including Native healing, often have more success with chronic stress-related diseases than allopathic medicine, which is most successful with what has been called "heroic" medicine—medical intervention with high-powered drugs, surgical procedures, or genetic manipulation. This raises the interesting question of why traditional therapies are successful with chronic diseases.

According to Russell Willier, an individual is composed of three elements: physical, emotional, and spiritual. Illness upsets the internal balance of these elements and thus has spiritual, psychological, and physiological manifestations. Regardless of the etiology of an illness, treatment must address itself to all three of these elements. In other words, treatment must be holistic and must be administered not by a specialist in one of these three dimensions, but by a practitioner who understands the relations among the elements involved. The healer must simultaneously be a medicine man, a psychologist, and a priest or shaman. On occasion, the additional role of performer is added. He must know a great deal about plants; must know the rituals that open windows between the human and spiritual worlds; must know diseases and whether or not he can treat them; and must know how to put both himself and the patient in the right frame of mind so spiritual power can flow in to assist the medicine in restoring a proper balance and to effect a cure.

Many illnesses are psychosomatic in the sense of involving both mind and body. Perhaps psycho-spiritual-somatic is a more accurate description of the relationship. Russell Willier is quick to admit to the role of the well-known placebo effect, but he does not view this in a negative way. Faith alone is inadequate, as is the pharmacological effect of the medicine by itself. Because illness has psychological, spiritual, and somatic effects, treatment must address all these levels. I have often been asked how much of the healing by Native healers is due to the herbs, how much to psychological factors, and how much to spiritual factors. I reply that it is impossible to assign such percentages, as healing is due to the synergistic effect of all of these factors combined. In brief, Russell's treatment is not an example of faith healing. Nor is it an example of Native pharmacology. Rather, it is a complex blend of science, psychology, and religion in which both healer and patient must play an active role.

These principles can be illustrated in reference to the sweat lodge ceremony. For a "sweat," rocks are heated and placed in a pit in the middle of a frame made of willow bows and covered with canvas. Patients sit around the pit, the door flap is closed, and there is complete darkness. As the heat begins to build, patients must concentrate on their skin temperatures to avoid being burned. This provides mental focus and eliminates being distracted by thoughts about the past or plans for the future. The heat also releases salicylic acid, the main ingredient in aspirin, from the boughs that make up the sweat lodge. Periodically, the healer dips a branch in a pail of medicated water and sprinkles the water on the hot rocks to create a blast of medicated steam that fills the lodge and penetrates the towels and loose garments worn by the patients. The healer chants to the accompaniment of rattles, sings, and prays. He also talks about the importance of having faith and reassures patients that they will get well if they believe. Gradually, minds shift from a left-brain orientation to a right-brain orientation in which information, energy, and healing power are able to rise from the depths of the unconscious and penetrate the conscious mind. Patients may hear the voices of people, animals, and birds, and perhaps see the forms of spirits who serve as intermediaries between the spiritual and human worlds. Some people report seeing a ball of light move from the healer to the patients, one by one.

One round lasts about half an hour, after which the door flap is opened and cool air is allowed to enter. Following the break, the door is closed again and the second round begins. A sweat usually consists of four rounds in all. In some rounds, patients are encouraged to join in the singing of traditional songs and to participate in a pipe ceremony in which the pipe is passed around the circle in a clockwise direction. By the end of the ceremony, the medicated water in the pail is gone, and patients emerge to sit around a fire and talk about the things that they heard and saw in the ceremony. Food offerings are scraped into the fire, and everyone refreshes themselves with food and drink. Finally, thanks are given to the healer, and patients present him or her with any gifts they might have brought. Tired but relaxed, patients get dressed and silently return home.

Native healing has the potential to help individuals from all ethnic groups, but it cannot be easily institutionalized. Interaction with a healer is intensive and personal, and requires commitment. For example, a patient may have to travel hundreds of miles to visit the healer and make a request for help, accompanied by a gift of tobacco and colored cloths or ribbons that are hung in the sweat lodge. The patient may then have to wait several days while the healer meditates in the forest to obtain advice concerning how to treat the patient, what herbs to combine, and where to find the herbs. The healer might receive a message that the patient should immediately be referred to a medical doctor or sent to the hospital. The greater the commitment on the part of the patient, the better the results usually are.

After I have talked to medical practitioners and showed slides of patients who have improved under Russell Willier's care, physicians in the audience sometimes ask if they can refer their patients to Russell or if they can obtain some of the medicines he uses. This usually is not possible, as only a limited number of people can be accommodated in a sweat lodge ceremony, and herbal combinations may not be effective unless used in a ritual setting that encourages participation and faith on the part of the patient. A ceremony such as a sweat is a drama in which shaman, patients, and spirits all become actors in a way that encourages emotional and psychological involvement because, unless the whole person is involved, chronic stress-related diseases are not likely to be helped.

Russell Willier is quick to admit that rattles and chants are designed to partially hypnotize a person and put him or her in a suggestible state of mind in which suggestions from the healer can trigger the mind to command the brain, the immune system, and the hormonal system to create the energies and chemicals needed to effect a cure. Although there are limits to this kind of healing, there is a great deal of scope for curing a variety of diseases, including those caused by mental and spiritual problems.

A good deal of further research needs to be conducted on Native healing if its efficacy is to be firmly established. Ideally, this might involve setting up a clinic with one or more Native healers and a medical doctor, whose role would be to order the medical records for a patient to be treated by a Native healer. These records would be obtained both before and after treatment. The physician would also have the authority to order additional diagnostic measures that might be needed to assess the effectiveness of treatment, as well as to intervene if the patient had an adverse reaction to a medicine or treatment. If enough such "case studies" were compiled for a variety of healers and if these results indicated which illnesses can be effectively treated with Native healing, the medical profession might be more willing to cooperate with Native healers to better address the health problems of modern, ethnically diverse societies. In complex societies in which health care costs are spiraling out of control, it is important to consider ways of combining traditional and modern healing practices in a complementary approach in which modern medicine with its high-tech approach is used to address problems that require fast, heroic measures, while traditional practitioners take care of chronic stress-related diseases that require a more personal approach. It is hoped that this book is one step in that direction.

Conclusion

This book is a historic document in that it is, to the best of our knowledge, the first time that a Native healer has agreed to share in writing his or her repertoire of herbal medicines and where they are found. This is the culmination of a long process, beginning in the 1980s when Russell Willier had the courage to begin sharing his knowledge in the hope that a book on the topic (*Cry of the Eagle: Encounters with a Cree Healer*) might inspire Native young people to become interested in traditional Native culture, spirituality, and healing. He also hoped that demonstrating the effectiveness of Native medicine would help preserve it for the future and help pave the way for greater cooperation between Native healers and Western medical practitioners in the interests of improving health care.

At first, Russell Willier was criticized for sharing this knowledge, but over the years, other healers began to realize that there is a real danger that much traditional knowledge could die out as the elders pass on. Today, there is widespread support for recording knowledge of medicinal plants and how they are used for future generations. The Centre for the Cross-Cultural Study of Health and Healing (now the Centre for Health and Culture) at the University of Alberta, with the help of the director, Dr. Earle Waugh, and Clifford Cardinal, a prominent Native healer on staff, is spearheading an effort to document the medicinal knowledge of a number of Native healers across Canada. The task ahead is a challenging one, as there are numerous Native healers with priceless knowledge. It is not a matter of simply choosing a prominent healer from each cultural group, as different healers within the same group possess different knowledge that has been passed down to them from sacred traditions with considerable antiquity. Thus it may be necessary in some cases to include more than one individual from a cultural group. Other sources of variation in traditional medicinal knowledge include things like differing histories of cultural repression and differing geographical climates.

As the task progresses, however, a solid base of traditional medicinal knowledge will gradually be established to provide a foundation for future cultural revitalization, training of young healers, and education of aboriginals and others in medical schools. The database will also provide a foundation for conducting scientific investigations of the efficacy of Native medicine, how this efficacy can be explained, and how this knowledge can be used to broaden and increase the efficacy of health care systems as a whole. It is important to emphasize that future books on this topic will not reveal complex medicinal formulas that are intended to be used in a ritual context. This kind of sacred knowledge must continue to be safeguarded by healers and scientists alike to prevent it from falling into the hands of those who wish to use it for profit. Rather, future books will provide a valuable resource for aboriginal healers and elders who wish to instruct young people on what the traditional herbs look like and where they can be found. Instruction concerning how to combine the herbs into medicines and how to use these medicines properly must continue to be provided by qualified healers.

Appendix A

Maps of Areas
Where Willier Collects His Herbs

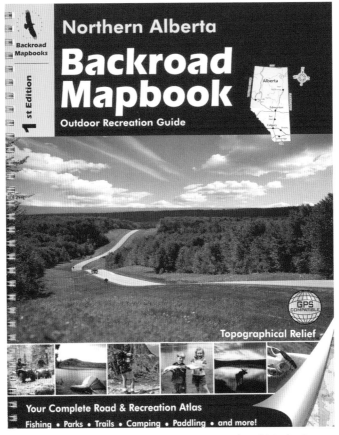

Backroad Mapbook cover

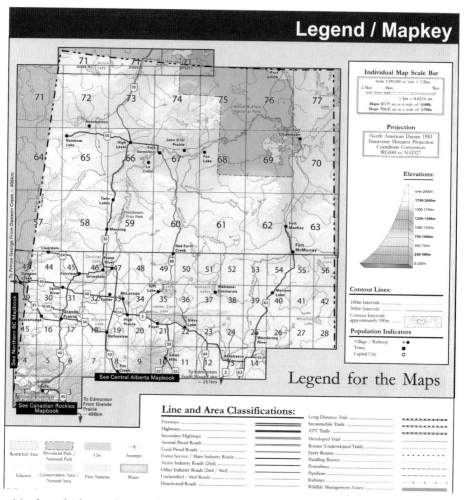

Map legend. The numbers on this legend correspond to the larger maps shown on the following pages. The legend shows the location of each of the larger maps in relation to the broader context. Only a portion of each of the larger maps is reproduced, which is why they do not exactly match the map legend.

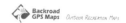

Areas in Northern Alberta Where Russell Willier and Other Native Healers Pick Medicinal Herbs

Note: The names of the plants are the names used by Willier

Map Page # (corresponds to #s on map, page IX)	General Area (nearest town)	Herbs Picked
2,3,4,5	Grande Cache	Small Arrow Sweet Pine
8	Fox Creek	Small Arrow Rat Smell Root Rat Root Yellow Pond Lilly
9	Fox Creek and Swan Hills	Small Arrow Big Arrow Balsam Poplar
10	Swan Hills	Yellow Pond Lilly
15	Beaverlodge	Yellow Pond Lilly
19	Valley View	Rat Smell Root
20	High Prairie	Diamond Willow Fungus Big Arrow Yellow Pond Lilly
21	Faust	Rat Small Root Big Arrow
22	Slave Lake	Frog Pants Pitcher Plant
23	Slave Lake	Big Arrow Yellow Pond Lilly
29	Dawson Creek, B.C.	Small Arrow Tamarack Birch Balsam Poplar
30	Spirit River	Diamond Willow Fungus
34, 35, 36	Area north of Lesser Slave Lake	Rat Root Seneca Snakeroot Gum Flower Rabbit Root Small Arrow Big Arrow Yellow Pond Lilly
46	Grimshaw	Same as above (pp 34-36) Diamond Willow Fungus
49	Gift Lake	Small Arrow Big Arrow Yellow Pond Lilly
58	Manning	Small Arrow Yellow Pond Lilly
59	Manning	Morning Flower Diamond Willow Fungus

Key

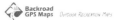

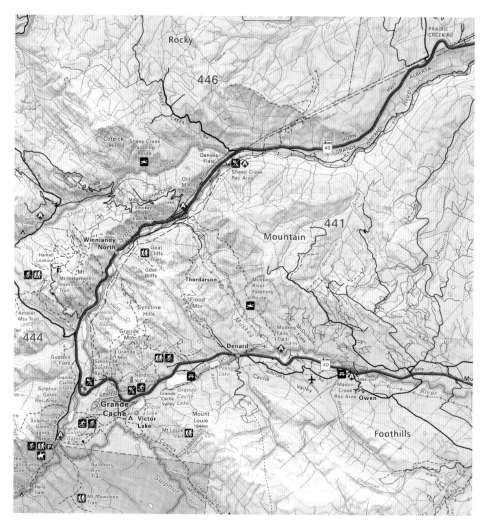

Map 2

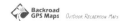

Backroad GPS Maps *Outdoor Recreation Maps*

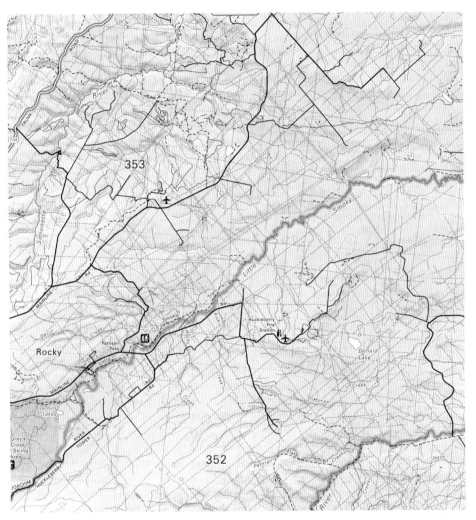

Map 3

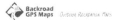

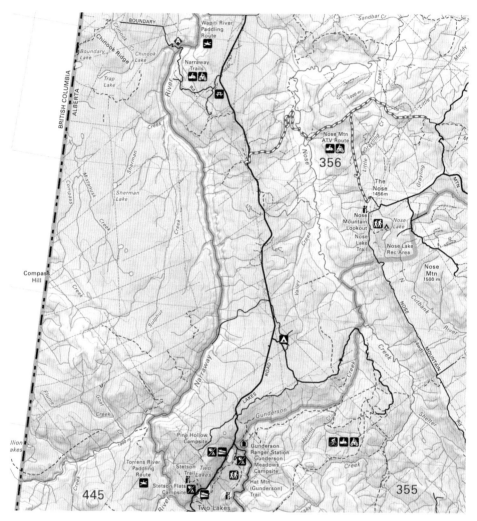

Map 4

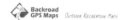

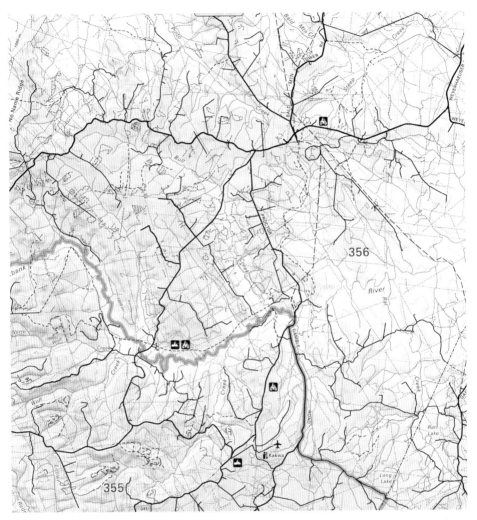

Map 5

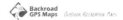

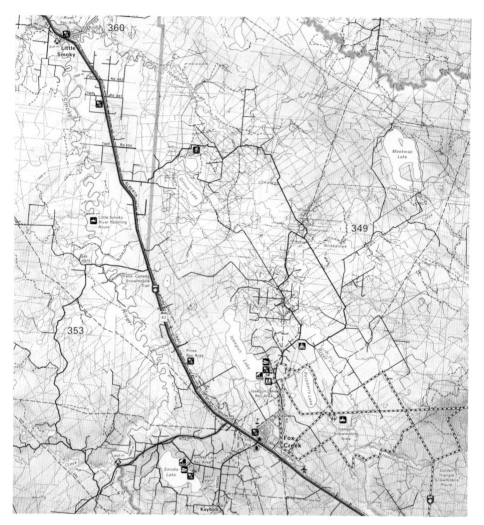

Map 8

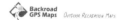

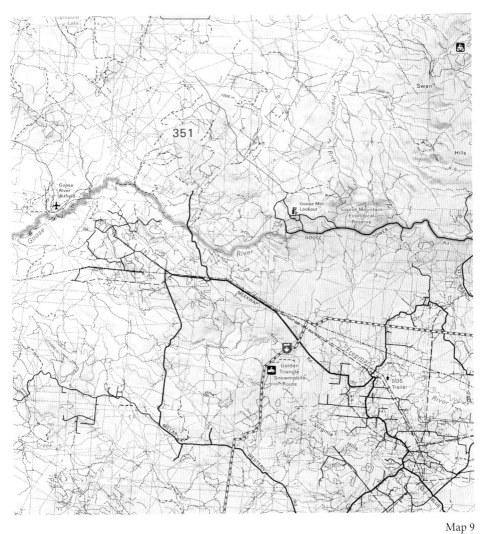

Map 9

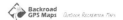

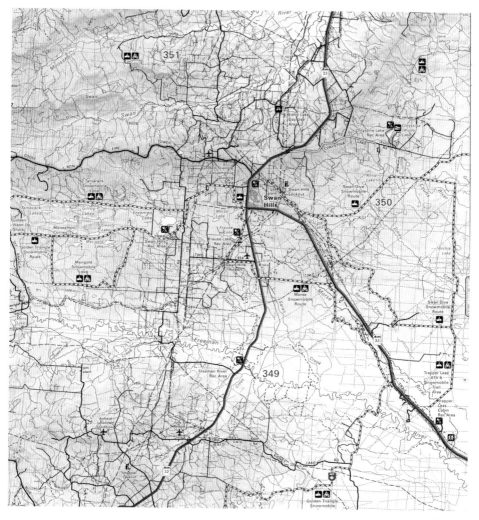

Map 10

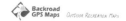

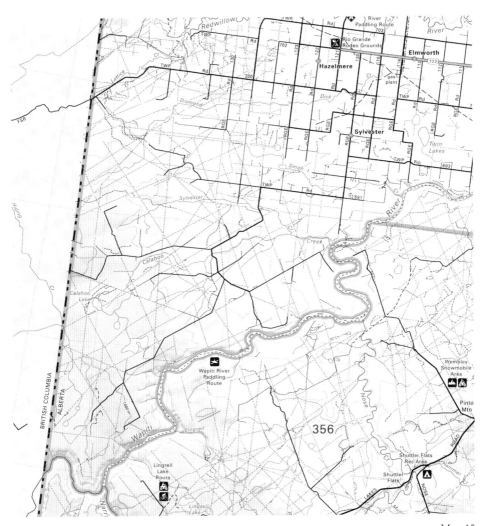

Map 15

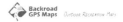

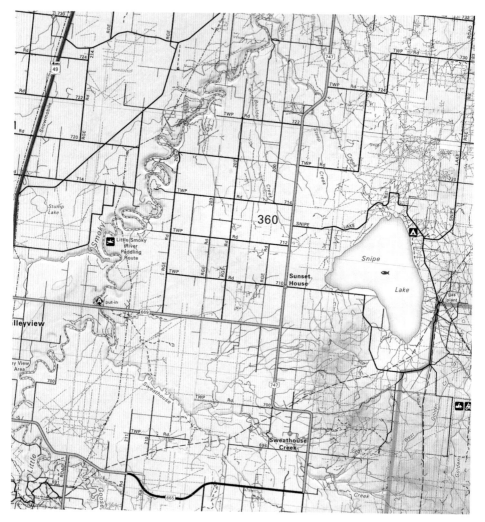

Map 19

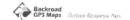

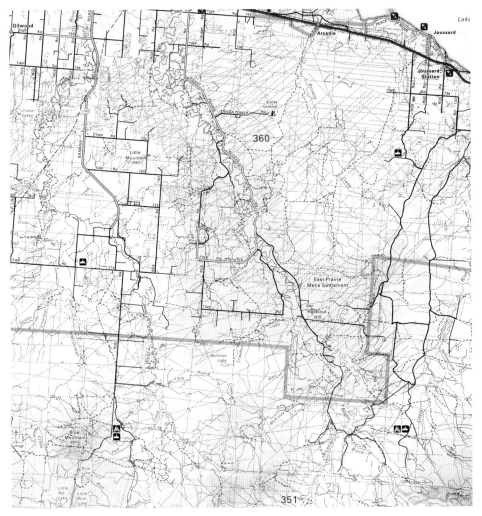

Map 20

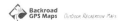

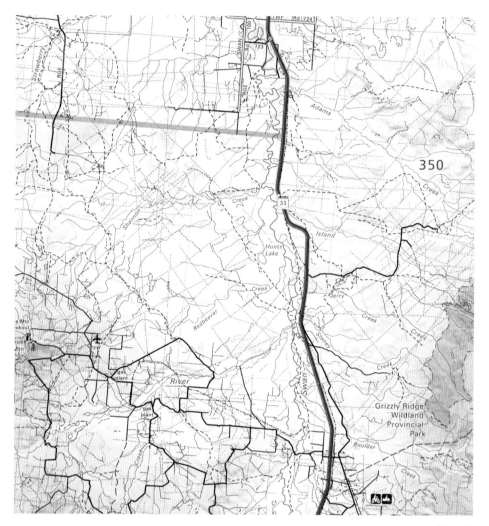

Map 21

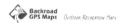

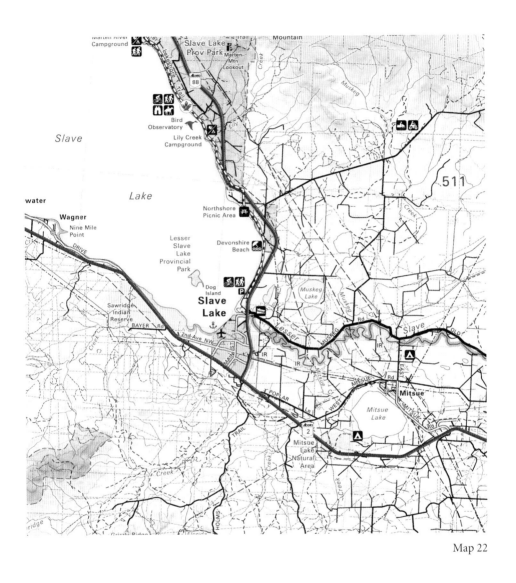

Map 22

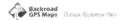

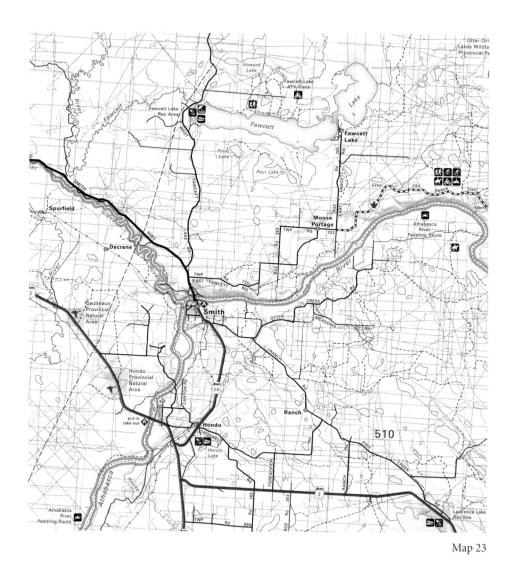

Map 23

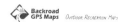

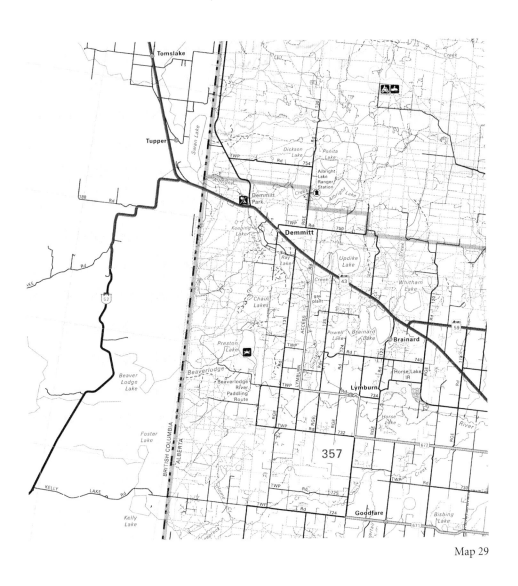

Map 29

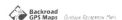

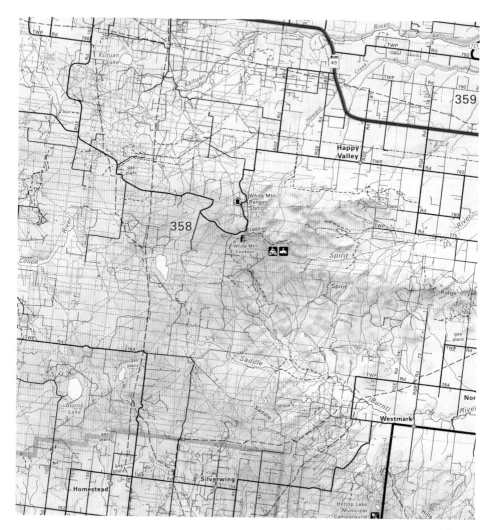

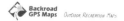

Map 30

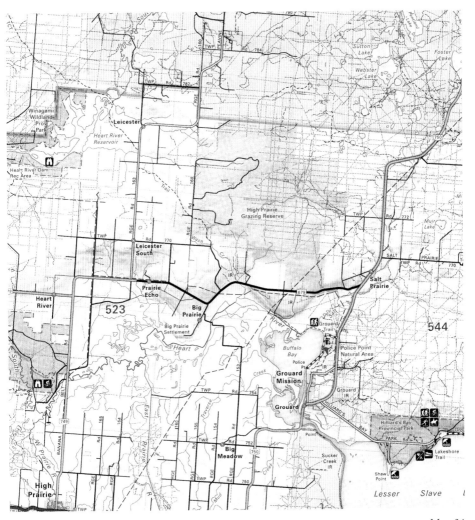

Map 34

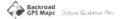

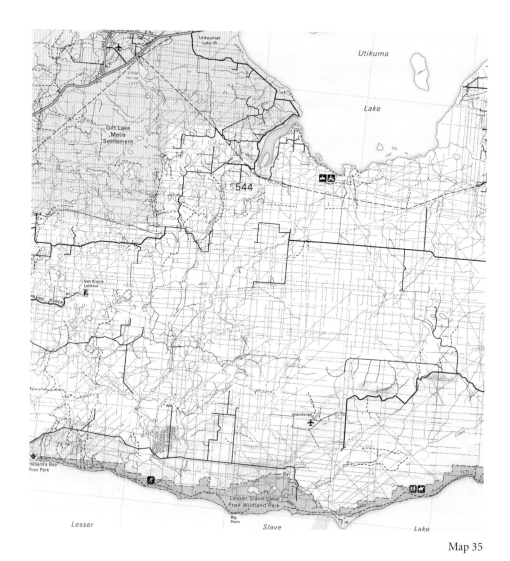

Map 35

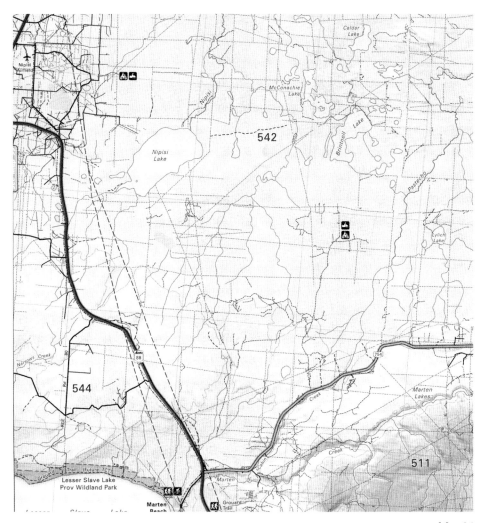

Map 36

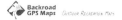

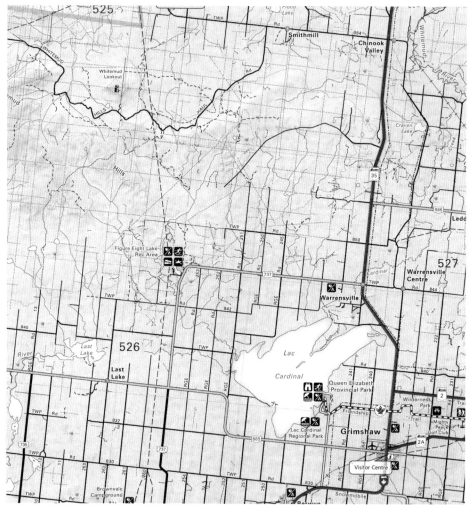

Map 46

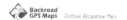

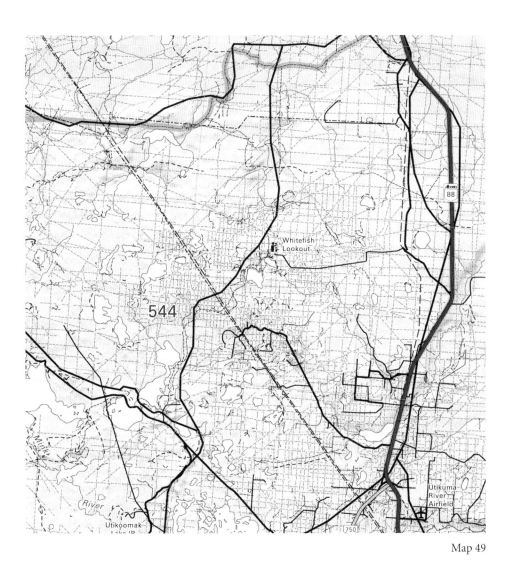

Map 49

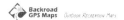

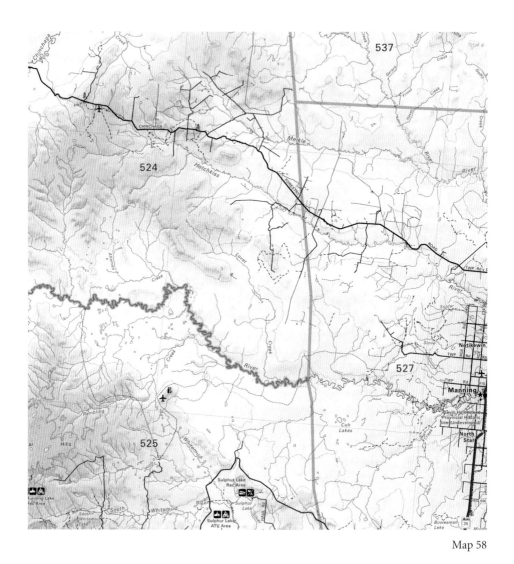

Map 58

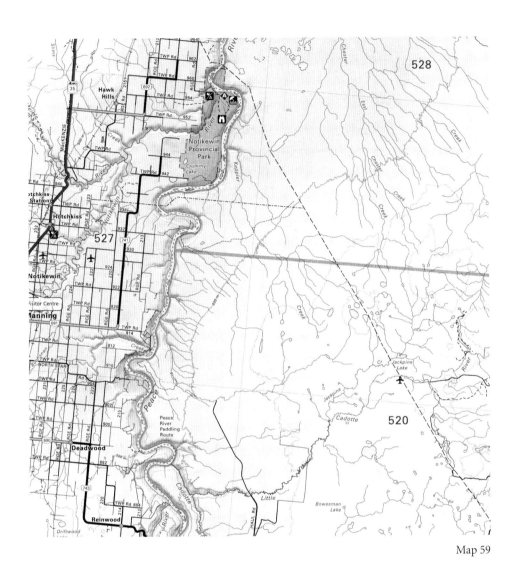

Map 59

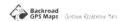

Appendix B

Index of Common English Names for the Plants Used by Willier

Appendix C

Index of Cree Names for the Plants Used by Willier

Appendix D

Index of English Names Used by Willier for the Plants He Uses

References

Acuña, U. M., D. E. Atha, J. Ma, M. H. Nee, and E. J. Kennelly. "Antioxidant Capacities of Ten Edible North American Plants." *Phytotherapy Research* 16, no. 1 (2002): 63–65.

Applequist, Wendy, and Daniel E. Moerman. "Yarrow (*Achillea millefolium* L.): A Neglected Panacea? A Review of Ethnobotany, Bioactivity, and Biochemical Research." *Economic Botany* 65, no. 2 (2011): 207–23.

Baldea, N., L. A. Martineau, et al. "Inhibition of Intestinal Glucose Absorption by Anti-Diabetic Medicinal Plants Derived from the James Bay Cree Traditional Pharmacopeia." *Journal of Ethnopharmacology* 132, no. 2 (2010): 473–82.

Belaiche, P., and O. Lievoux. "Clinical Studies on the Palliative Treatment of Prostatic Adenoma with Extract of Urtica Root." *Phytotherapy Research* 5 (1991): 267–269.

Beresford-Kroeger, Diana. *Arboretum Borealis: A Lifeline of the Planet.* Ann Arbor: University of Michigan Press, 2010.

Brinker, Francis. *Herb Contraindications and Drug Interactions.* 3rd ed. Sandy, OR: Eclectic Medical Publications, 2001.

Candan, M., M. Yilmaz, T. Tay, M. Erdem, and A. O. Turk. "Antimicrobial Activity of Extracts of the Lichen *Parmelia sulcata* and Its Salazinic Acid Constituent." *Zeitschrift für Naturforschung C: A Journal of Biosciences* 62, no. 7 (2007): 619–21.

Clare, B. A., R. S. Conroy, and K. Spelman. "The Diuretic Effect in Human Subjects of an Extract of *Taraxacum officinale* Folium over a Single Day." *Journal of Alternative and Complementary Medicine* 15, no. 8 (2009): 929–34.

Cook, W. H. *The Physio-Medical Dispensatory: A Treatise on Therapeutics, Materia Medica, and Pharmacy in Accordance with the Principles of Physiological Medication.* Cincinnati, OH: William Cook, 1869.

Coutinho, H., J. Costa, O. Edeltrudes, et al. "Potentiating Effect of Mentha arvensis and Chlorpromazine in the Resistance to Aminoglycosides of Methicillin-Resistant Staphylococcus aureus." *Vivo* 23, no. 2 (2009): 287–89.

Dall'Acqua, S., R. M. Gaion, C. Bolego, A. Cignarella, and G. Innocenti. "Vasoprotective Activity of Standardized *Achillea millefolium* Extract." *Phytomedicine* 18, no. 12 (2011): 1031–36.

Dufour, D., A. Pichette, et al. "Antioxidant, Anti-inflammatory and Anticancer Activities of Methanolic Extracts from *Ledum groenlandicum*." *Journal of Ethnopharmacology* 111 (2007): 22–28.

Ellingwood, F. *American Materia Medica, Therapeutics and Pharmacognosy*. Whitefish, MT: Kessinger, 1915, republished 2010.

Fraser, M. H., A. Cuerrier, P. Haddad, J. T. Arnason, P. Owen, and T. Johns. "Medicinal Plants of Cree Communities (Quebec, Canada): Antioxidant Activity of Plants Used to Treat Type 2 Diabetes Symptoms." *Canadian Journal of Physiology and Pharmacology* 58, no. 11 (2007): 1200–1204.

Frejnagel, S. S., and Z. Zdunczyk. "Chokeberry Polyphenols Reduce Prooxidative Influence of Oxidized Fats in Rats' Diets." *Polish Journal of Veterinary Sciences* 11, no. 2 (2008): 125–32.

Fulda, Simone. "Betulinic Acid for Cancer Treatment and Prevention." *International Journal of Molecular Sciences* 9, no. 6 (2008): 1098–1107.

García-Pérez, M. E., M. Royer, A. Duque-Fernandez, P. N. Diouf, T. Stevanovic, and R. Pouliot. "Antioxidant, Toxicological and Antiproliferative Properties of Canadian Polyphenolic Extracts on Normal and Psoriatic Keratinocytes." *Journal of Ethnopharmacology* 132, no. 1 (2010): 251–58.

Gescher, K., and A. M. Deters. "*Typha latifolia* L. Fruit Polysaccharides Induce the Differentiation and Stimulate the Proliferation of Human Keratinocytes In Vitro." *Journal of Ethnopharmacology* 137, no. 1 (2011): 352–58.

Gilani, A., A. J. Shah, M. Ahmad, and F. Shaheen. "Antispasmodic Effect of *Acorus calamus* Linn. Is Mediated Through Calcium Channel Blockade." *Phytotherapy Research* 20, no. 12 (2006): 1080–84.

Han, S., Z. Li, Y. Li, and R. Zhong. "Antitumor Effect of the Extract of

Birch Bark and Its Influence to the Immune Function." *Zhong Yao Cai* 23, no. 6 (2000): 343–45.

Harbilas, D., L. C. Martineau, C. S. Harris, D. Spoor, et al. "Evaluation of the Antidiabetic Potential of Selected Medicinal Plant Extracts from the Canadian Boreal Forest Used to Treat Symptoms of Diabetes: Part II." *Canadian Journal of Physiology and Pharmacology* 87, no. 6 (2009): 479–92.

Harbilas, D., D. Vallerand, A. Brault, A. Saleem, J. Arneson, L. Musallam, and P. Haddad. "*Larix laricina,* an Antidiabetic Alternative Treatment from the Cree of Northern Quebec Pharmacopoeia, Decreases Glycemia and Improves Insulin Sensitivity *In Vivo.*" *Evidence-Based Complementary and Alternative Medicine,* article ID 296432, 2012.

Harbilas, D., D. Vallerand, A. Brault, A. Saleem, J. Arneson, L. Musallam, and P. Haddad. "*Populus balsamifera* Extract and Its Active Component Salicortin Reduce Obesity and Attenuate Insulin Resistance in a Diet-Induced Obese Mouse Model." *Evidence-Based Complementary and Alternative Medicine,* article ID 172537, 2013.

Harmala, P., S. Kaltia, H. Vuorela, and R. Hiltunen. "A Furanocoumarin from *Angelica archangelica.*" *Planta Medica* 58, no. 3 (1991): 287–89.

Harris, C. S., A. Muhammad, A. Saleem, P. Haddad, J. T. Arnason, and S. Bennett. "Characterizing the Cytoprotective Activity of *Sarracenia purpurea* L., a Medicinal Plant That Inhibits Glucotoxicity in PC12 Cells." *BMC Complementary and Alternative Medicine* 12 (2012): 245.

Kashiwada, Y., H. K. Wang, T. Nagao, et al. "Anti-AIDS Agents. 30. Anti-HIV Activity of Oleanolic Acid, Pomolic Acid, and Structurally Related Triterpenoids." *Journal of Natural Products* 61, no. 9 (1998): 1090–95.

Keane, Kahlee. The Standing People: Field Guide of Medicinal Plants for the Prairie Provinces. Saskatoon, Saskatchewan: Root Woman and Dave, 2012.

Keane, Kahlee, and Dave Howarth. *The Standing People.* Saskatoon, Saskatchewan: Root Woman and Dave, 2003.

Keller, K., K. P. Odenthal, and E. Leng-Peschlow. "Spasmolytische Wirkung des Isoasaronfreien Kalmus." *Planta Medica* 51, no. 1 (1985): 6–9.

Kiss, A., J. Kowalski, and M. F. Melzig. "Compounds from Epilobium angustifolium Inhibit the Specific Metallopeptidases ACE, NEP and APN." *Planta Medica* 70, no. 10 (2004): 919–23.

Ko, F. N., T. S. Wu, M. J. Liou, T. F. Huang, and C. M. Teng. "Vasorelaxation of Rat Thoracic Aorta Caused by Osthole Isolated from *Angelica pubescens*." *European Journal of Pharmacology* 219, no. 1 (1992): 29–34.

Kraft, T., M. Dey, R. B. Rogers, D. M. Ribnicky, D. M. Gipp, W. T. Cefalu, I. Raskin, and M. A. Lila. "Phytochemical Composition and Metabolic Performance-Enhancing Activity of Dietary Berries Traditionally Used by Native North Americans." *Journal of Agricultural and Food Chemistry* 56, no. 3 (2008): 654–60.

Leacock, Stephen. *Adventures of the Far North: A Chronicle of the Arctic Seas.* Vol. 20 of The Chronicles of Canada. Whitefish, MT: Kessinger, [1920] 2009.

LeClaire, Nancy, and George Cardinal. *Alberta Elders' Cree Dictionary.* Edited by Earle Waugh. Edmonton, Alberta: University of Alberta Press and Duval House, 1998.

Martineau, L. C., D. C. A. Adeyiwola-Spoor, D. Vallerand, et al. "Enhancement of Muscle Cell Glucose Uptake by Medicinal Plant Species of Canada's Native Populations Is Mediated by a Common, Metformin-like Mechanism." *Journal of Ethnopharmacology* 127, no. 2 (2010): 396–406.

Martineau, L. C., J. Hervé, A. Muhamad, et al. "Anti-Adipogenic Activities of *Alnus incana* and *Populus balsamifera* Bark Extracts, Part I: Sites and Mechanisms of Action." *Planta Medica* 76, no. 13 (2010): 1439–46.

Mazzio, Elizabeth, and K. Soliman. "*In Vitro* Screening for the Tumoricidal Properties of International Medicinal Herbs." *Phytotherapy Research* 23, no. 3 (2009): 385–98.

McCune, L. M., and T. Johns. "Antioxidant Activity in Medicinal Plants Associated with the Symptoms of Diabetes Mellitus Used by the Indigenous Peoples of the North American Boreal Forest." *Journal of Ethnopharmacology* 82 (2002): 197–205.

McCutcheon, A. R., S. M. Ellis, R. E. W. Hancock, and G. H. N. Towers. "Antibiotic Screening of Medicinal Plants of the British Columbian Native Peoples." *Journal of Ethnopharmacology* 37, no. 3 (1992): 213–23.

McCutcheon, A. R., S. M. Ellis, R. E. W. Hancock, and G. H. N. Towers. "Antifungal Screening of Medicinal Plants of British Columbian Native Peoples." *Journal of Ethnopharmacology* 44, no. 3 (1994): 157–69.

McCutcheon, A. R., T. E. Roberts, E. Gibbons, S. M. Ellis, L. A. Babiuk, R. E. W. Hancock, and G. Towers. "Antiviral Screening of British Columbian Medicinal Plants." *Journal of Ethnopharmacology* 49 (1995): 101–10.

McFarlin, B. L., M. H. Gibson, J. O'Rear, and P. Harman. "A National Survey of Herbal Preparation Use by Nurse-Midwives for Labor Stimulation: Review of the Literature and Recommendations for Practice." *Journal of Nurse-Midwifery* 44, no. 3 (1999): 205–16.

Moore, Michael. *Medicinal Plants of the Desert and Canyon West.* Santa Fe: Museum of New Mexico Press, 1989.

Muceniece, R., K. Saleniece, J. Rumaks, et al. "Betulin Binds to Gamma-Aminobutyric Acid Receptors and Exerts Anticonvulsant Action in Mice." *Pharmacology Biochemistry Behavior* 90, no. 4 (2008): 712–16.

Muhammad, A., J. A. Guerrero-Anaico, L. C. Martineau, et al. "Antidiabetic Compounds from *Sarracenia purpurea* Used Traditionally by the Eeyou Istchee Cree First Nation." *Journal of Natural Products* 75, no. 7 (2012): 1284–88.

Müller-Jakic, B., W. Breu, A. Pröbstle, K. Redl, H. Greger, and R. Bauer. "In Vitro Inhibition of Cyclooxygenase and 5-lipoxygenase by Alkamides from Echinacea and Achillea Species." *Planta Medica* 60, no. 1 (1994): 37–40.

Nan Shang, B. Walshe-Roussel, A. Muhammed, L. Musallam, A. Saleem, J. Arnason, A. Cuerrier, J. Guerrero-Analco, and P. Haddad. "Adipogenic Constituents from the Bark of *Larix laricina,* an Important Medicinal Plant Used Traditionally by the Cree of Eeyou Istchee (Quebec, Canada) for the Treatment of Type 2 Diabetes Symptoms." *Journal of Ethnopharmacology* 141, no. 3 (2012): 1051–57.

Nishizawa, K., I. Nakata, A. Kishida, W. Ayer, and L. M. Browne. "Some Biologically Active Tannins of *Nuphar variegatum.*" *Phytochemistry* 29, no. 8 (1990): 2491–94.

Owen, P., and T. Johns. "Xanthine Oxidase Inhibitory Activity of Northeastern North American Plant Remedies Used for Gout." *Journal of Ethnopharmacology* 64, no. 2 (1999): 149–60.

Painter, T. J. "Concerning the Wound-Healing Properties of Sphagnum Holocellulose: The Maillard Reaction in Pharmacology." *Journal of Ethnopharmacology* 88, nos. 2–3 (2003): 145–48.

Panizzi, L., S. Catalano, C. Miarelli, P. L. Cioni, and E. Campeol. "In Vitro Antimicrobial Activity of Extracts and Isolated Constituents of *Geum rivale*." *Phytotherapy Research* 14, no. 7 (2000): 561–63.

Parsons, M., M. Simpson, and T. Ponton. "Raspberry Leaf and Its Effect on Labour: Safety and Efficacy." *Australian College of Midwives Journal* 12, no. 3 (1999): 20–25.

Phillips, Charles D. F. *Materia Medica and Therapeutics.* New York: W. Wood, 1879.

Pukalskas, A., T. A. van Beek, et al. "Identification of Radical Scavengers in Sweet Grass (*Hierchloe odorata*)." *Journal of Agricultural and Food Chemistry* 50, no. 10 (2002): 214–19.

Qi, Z., J. Xue, Y. Zhang, H. Want, M. Xie. "Osthole Ameliorates Insulin Resistance by Increment of Adiponectin Release in High-Fat and High-Sucrose-Induced Fatty Liver Rats." *Planta Medica* 77, no. 3 (2011): 231–35.

Rankovic, B., M. Misic, and M. Sukdolak. "Evaluation of Antimicrobial Activity of the Lichens *Lasallia pustulata, Parmelia sulcata, Umbilicaria crustulosa* and *Umbilicaria cylindrical*." *Mikrobiologya* 76, no. 6 (2007): 817–21.

Rezvani, M. E., A. Roohbakhsh, M. Allahtovakoli, and A. Shamsizadeh. "Anticonvulsant Effect of Aqueous Extract of *Valeriana officinalis* in Amygdala-Kindled Rats: Possible Involvement of Adenosine." *Journal of Ethnopharmacology* 127 (2010): 313–18.

Ribnicky, D. M., A. Poulev, and I. Raskin. "The Determination of Salicylates in *Gaultheria procumbens* for Use as a Natural Aspirin Alternative." *Journal of Nutraceuticals, Functional and Medical Foods* 4, no. 1 (2003): 39–51.

Richardson, John. *Wacousta: A Tale of the Canadas.* Toronto, Ontario: McClelland and Stewart, [1832] 1991.

Rogers, Robert Dale. *Rogers' Herbal Manual.* Wildwood, Alberta: Karamat Wilderness Ways, 2000.

Rogers, Robert Dale. *Herbal–Drug Interactions.* Edmonton, Alberta: Capital Health, 2003.

Rogers, Robert Dale. *The Fungal Pharmacy: The Complete Guide to Medicinal Mushrooms and Lichens of North America.* Berkeley, CA: North Atlantic Books, 2011.

Rogers, Robert Dale. *Rogers' School of Herbal Medicine*, Vols. 1–15. Edmonton, Alberta: Prairie Deva Press, 2014.

Roschek, B., Jr., R. C. Fink, M. McMichael, and R. S. Alberte. "Nettle Extract (*Urtica dioica*) Affects Key Receptors and Enzymes Associated with Allergic Rhinitis." *Phytotherapy Research* 23, no. 7 (2009): 920–26.

Rose, Kiva. "River Medicine: Alder's Transformation of Lymph, Blood, and The Human Ecology." www.bearmedicineherbals.com/river medicine.html, January 5, 2012.

Salikhova, R. A., and G. G. Poroshenko. "Antimutagenic Properties of Angelica archangelica L." *Vestnik Rossiĭskoĭ Akademii Meditsinskikh Nauk* 1 (1995): 58–61.

Salisbury, E. J. *Weeds and Aliens.* #43 New Naturalist Series. London: Collins, 1961.

Schwarz, A. "Beethoven's Renal Disease Based on His Autopsy: A Case of Papillary Necrosis." *American Journal of Kidney Diseases* 21, no. 6 (1993): 643–52.

Sheh Meng Lan, Pu Su, and Ze Hui Pan. "The Comparative Study of Pollen Morphology of Angelica L. Between East Asia and North America." *Journal of Plant Resources and Environment* 6, no. 1 (1997): 41–47.

Shikov, A. N., G. I. Diachuk, D. V. Sergeev, O. N. Pozharitskaya, E. V. Esaulenko, V. M. Kosman, and V. G. Makarov. "Birch Bark Extract as Therapy for Chronic Hepatitis C—a Pilot Study." *Phytomedicine* 18, no. 10 (2011): 807–10.

Simpson, M., M. Parsons, J. Greenwood, and K. Wade. "Raspberry Leaf in Pregnancy: Its Safety and Efficacy in Labor." *Journal of Midwifery and Women's Health* 46, no. 2 (2001): 51–59.

Spoor, D. C. A., L. C. Martineau, C. Leduc, et al. "Selected Plant Species from the Cree Pharmacopocia of Northern Quebec Possess Anti-Diabetic Potential." *Canadian Journal of Physiology and Pharmacology* 84, nos. 8–9 (2006): 847–58.

Tucker, A., and L. Chambers. "*Mentha canadensis* L. (Lamiaceae): A Relict Amphidiploid from the Lower Tertiary." *Taxon* 51, no. 4 (2002): 703–18.

Verma, N., B. C. Behera, and B. O. Sharma. "Glucosidase Inhibitory and Radical Scavenging Properties of Lichen Metabolites Salazinic Acid, Sekikaic Acid and Usnic Acid." *Hacettepe Journal of Biology and Chemistry* 401 (2012): 7–21.

Vianna, R., A. Brault, L. C. Martineau, R. Couture, J. Arnason, P. S. Haddad. "In Vivo Anti-Diabetic Activity of the Ethanolic Crude Extract of Sorbus decora C. K. Schneid. (Rosacea): A Medicinal Plant Used by Canadian James Bay Cree Nations to Treat Symptoms Related to Diabetes." *Evid Based Complement Alternat Med 2011* (2011): 237941.

Vitali, F., G. Fonte, A. Saija, and B. Tita. "Inhibition of Intestinal Motility and Secretion of Extracts of Epilobium spp. in Mice." *Journal of Ethnopharmacology* 107, no. 3 (2006): 342–48.

Vuorela, H., P. Vuorela, K. Tornquist, and S. Alaranta. "Calcium Channel Blocking Activity: Screening Methods for Plant Derived Compounds." *Phytomedicine* 4, no. 2 (1997): 167–80.

Willey, L. B., S. P. Mady, D. J. Cobaugh, et al. "Valerian Overdose: A Case Report. *Veterinary and Human Toxicology* 37 (1995): 364–65.

Wood, Matthew. *The Book of Herbal Wisdom.* Berkeley, CA: North Atlantic Books, 1997.

Wood, Matthew. *The Earthwise Herbal: A Complete Guide to New World Medicinal Plants.* Berkeley, CA: North Atlantic Books, 2009.

Yang, G. Y., and W. Wang. "Clinical Studies on the Treatment of Coronary Heart Disease with *Valeriana officinalis*." *Chung Kuo Chung Hsi I Chieh Ho Tsa Chih* 41, no. 9 (1994): 540–42.

Young, David E. *The Mouse Woman of Gabriola: Brain, Mind, and Icon Interactions in Spontaneous Healing.* Gabriola, British Columbia: Coastal Tides Press, 2013.

Young, David E., Grant Ingram, and Lise Swartz. *Cry of the Eagle: Encounters with a Cree Healer.* Toronto, Ontario: University of Toronto Press, 1989.

Zhang, Y., Y. Cao, Q. Wang, L. Zheng, J. Zhang, and L. He. "A Potential Calcium Antagonist and Its Antihypertensive Effects." *Fitoterapia* 82, no. 7 (2011): 988–96.

Index

About the Authors

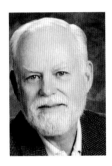

DAVID YOUNG spent much of his childhood in Sierra Leone, West Africa. After returning to the United States, he graduated with a BA in sociology and philosophy from the University of Indianapolis, followed by a BD in religion and anthropology from Yale University, an MA in Asian Studies from the East West Center, University of Hawaii, and a PhD in anthropology from Stanford University. Dr. Young taught anthropology for many years at the University of Alberta in Canada before retiring to take a teaching position at Kansai Gaidai University in Japan. He has conducted fieldwork in Mexico, Japan, China, and northern Canada. Dr. Young has coauthored several books including *Cry of the Eagle: Encounters with a Cree Healer; Being Changed by Cross-Cultural Encounters: the Anthropology of Extraordinary Experience;* and *The Mouse Woman of Gabriola: Brain, Mind and Icon Interactions in Spontaneous Healing.* He also has copublished books on Japanese art, gardens, and architecture with his wife, Michiko. Dr. Young and his wife are retired and live on the island of Gabriola, off the west coast of Canada.

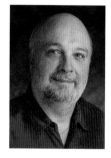

Robert Rogers (BSc, RH/AHG, FICN) has been a student of native plants and fungi from the Canadian prairies for more than forty years. He is a retired clinical herbalist, amateur mycologist, and professional member of the American Herbalist Guild. Rogers is an assistant clinical professor in family medicine at the University of Alberta. He has written more than twenty books and ebooks on the traditional use of plants and fungi of the boreal forest with special attention to application by aboriginal healers. Rogers teaches plant medicine at Grant MacEwan University and the Northern Star College of Mystical Studies in Edmonton and is a consultant to the herbal, mycological and nutraceutical industries, in addition to currently being chair of the medicinal mushroom committee of the North American Mycological Association, and being on the editorial board of the International Journal of Medicinal Mushrooms. Rogers lives in Edmonton, Canada, with his wife, Laurie. You can visit their webpage at www.self healdistributing.com.

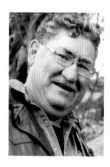

Russell Willier was born on the Sucker Creek Reserve in northern Alberta. He grew up in a large family of twelve brothers and sisters. His father was a skilled hunter and trapper who passed his knowledge about the traditional Woods Cree way of life on to his son. Willier attended Catholic mission school but quit in order to help his parents on the family farm. Even at an early age, he showed signs of having been selected by the Spirit World to be a healer, but he resisted for many years. Eventually, he accepted this responsibility and received the medicine bundle of his great grandfather, Moostoos, a well-known healer in the area and signer of Treaty 8. By the time Willier received his medicine bundle, the knowledge of how to use the little plant packets in his medicine bundle had been lost, so he showed them to elders and asked if they knew how these "combinations" were used. Gradually, over many years, he pieced together the information he needed to begin practice as a medicine man. Willier, who still lives on the Sucker Creek Reserve, travels extensively to treat those who call upon him for help.